I0105540

I LET IT GROW

Written by:
Sharon Domeny

I Let It Grow

Written By: Sharon Domeny
Edited By: Nalani Butler
Cover Design: Aaron C. Butler

ISBN: 9781967082391 (Paperback)
ISBN: 9781967082407 (eBook)

Library of Congress Control Number: 2025913175
2025 BookButler Publishing Company

All rights reserved. This book or any portion thereof may not be
reproduced in any form without permission from the copyright
holder, except as permitted by U.S. copyright law.

Printed in the United States of America

BookButler Publishing Company
Upper Marlboro, MD 20792
TheBookButler.com

BookButler Publishing Company titles may be purchased in bulk
for educational, business, fundraising, or sales promotional use.

For more information, please email: info@thebookbutler.com

BOOKBUTLER
PUBLISHING COMPANY

Dedication

This book is dedicated to all who have experienced the pain of generational trauma. I hope this book can help you bridge the gap of understanding those who pass it to us, how we experience it, and how we unknowingly pass it to the next generation. I also hope this is a book of healing. Healing that comes from true understanding and a determination to make the necessary changes to live wonderfully and fearlessly as your authentic self. In this way, I believe, the cycle will finally end. It didn't end with me, but my hope is that it will end with them.

In February of 2023, I decided to stop letting it grow.

Table of Contents

Introduction

In February of 2023, after nearly two decades of marriage, I left the man I promised God I would spend the rest of my life with. A friend of mine brought over a trailer, and I filled it with boxes of clothes and enough household items to get me started in my new apartment. All of the things we collected and created over the years, most of which stayed behind. My kids, both teenagers at the time, left with me— their stuff in the trailer right next to mine. I told my husband a few days before the move that I had leased an apartment and would be leaving. He was angry, but not surprised. Nobody was surprised. His business trip occupied him during the two days we spent packing. By the time he came home, the trailer was full. The next morning, we were gone.

It was surreal leaving everything. I looked at the house and the yard one last time before I left. The memories came flooding back. I could see the playset where my kids spent summers outside and the tree that held their first swing as babies. I visualized my daughter's big smile as I grabbed her toes when the swing moved her back to me. Now the yard was empty, holding nothing but these memories. I looked up at the window my son would look out when I came home, and then at the one my dog would excitedly jump in front of to welcome us back each night. This was my home. I remember waking up the day after we moved into that house, some seventeen years ago, looking out of my bedroom window, thinking about my baby that would soon be born and all the memories we would make. So much had changed since that day. One trailer and two cars full of our lives. Turns out you don't need much to start over.

Just a month earlier, I was on a pilgrimage in the Holy Land. I spent time in prayer while visiting Jerusalem, Nazareth, Bethlehem, and some of the holiest sites on earth. I prayed in the garden of Gethsemane and walked in the Jordan River. The trip was purposeful. I knew I was suffering, that my kids were suffering, and so was my marriage. Helpless, I looked for direction or perhaps even a sign from God himself. I spent time talking to my Priest. He shared scripture readings with me that allowed me to see that what I was experiencing in my home and marriage was not from God. I remember his exact words: "You cannot heal your husband; only God can do that." With the support of the Church, I felt I was making the right decision to leave.

By that time, things had gotten to a place where my husband and I barely tolerated each other. We lived in the same home, sure, but we rarely spoke. We had a large house and occupied different areas in it. Not even our bedroom held traces of us both, as I had moved out years before. Resentment and rage festered inside me over time, making it difficult to contain in our interactions, each laced with bitterness. I hated the person I was when I was around him. I hated *him*.

In therapy, I was told that my husband was emotionally abusive and that I was a victim of that abuse. My friends, many of whom were therapists, agreed. Books and videos echoed the same sentiment. It explained so much: my constant anxiety, my depressive episodes, my emotional struggles. I was also told that my husband was a narcissist. Looking back, I realize how easily that word is tossed around today. True narcissism is rare, but eager for answers at the time, I accepted the diagnosis without question.

Narcissists are often described as selfish, emotionally and financially abusive, lacking empathy, and having a desire for control. Many lie, cheat, have an inflated sense of self, and even struggle with substance use. Some of the traits fit my husband, but many did not. "No worries," my therapist assured me– he checked enough boxes to classify on the lower level of the narcissist spectrum. That was enough to justify my belief.

Two major emotions hit me when I learned that my husband might be a narcissist. First, I felt devastated. I mean, you pretty much learn that you have married and created life with a monster. It's a gut punch. I grieved for myself and my children. Then I felt.... relief. Maybe this was the reason my life had spiraled out of control. *He* was the problem. It validated my decision to leave.

But what I didn't realize then was how deeply my own confirmation bias shaped my thoughts. The truth is, we naturally seek out and remember information that reinforces our beliefs, while ignoring contradictory evidence. Once I was presented with the idea that my husband could be a narcissist, every unmet need, every inconsiderate and uncaring act, became proof of his flaws. I even kept a list to remind myself. The more I searched, the more I found, and it justified my rightness.

If your spouse is a narcissist, the common advice is clear: leave and never look back. Even the Catholic Church seemed to be on board with separation. I was told my only chance at healing was to cut ties completely. Narcissists don't have the capacity for love or emotional intimacy, nor do they desire it. He was broken and deficient beyond repair. I was the brave wife, charting a new life for myself and my children.

But this is not just a story of my husband's flaws. It is also a story of my own reflection. Part of my story is that I am a licensed clinical therapist myself. I'm trained at helping people unravel their problems, yet blind to my own. Sometimes it's easier to teach a principle than to apply it. Have you ever met a mechanic who drove around in an old beater car or a carpenter with a lot of unfinished "projects"? Same principle. I have added clinical information to this story because some of my healing was about applying what I already knew to my own life. Through my process of self-reflection and discovery, I gained insight and understanding into my own thoughts, belief systems, and behaviors. I began to see my role in the breakdown of our marriage. Yes, my husband was emotionally distant, self-serving, and unavailable. But that did not mean he was a full-blown narcissist hell bent on destruction. In fact, I realized we were more alike than I had ever admitted, just with different coping strategies.

Everyone I confided in only heard my side of the story. When I spoke about my experiences, I believed I was being honest, but I lacked a true understanding of my own patterns. Consequently, the advice I received was based on an incomplete, biased narrative. And while unhealthy dynamics were present in our marriage, I had to ask myself— did that absolve me of my own destructive behaviors?

I realized it did not. I was responsible for my actions, not just in this marriage but in every relationship I would ever have, including the one with myself. Since childhood, I had struggled with loneliness and a fear of intimacy that made it difficult to form secure attachments with people. I had always relied on others to "fix" me, yet nothing they gave ever felt like enough. It was time to learn how to give myself what I needed. It was time to heal.

Two years later, I return a better version of myself to share my story. Join me on this journey of self-reflection, where I learned to change the only person I could – myself. And bear in mind that you can too.

I let It Grow

Chapter 1

My Story

To truly understand the dynamics in my marriage, I had to look beyond the relationship itself to recognize how those toxic patterns developed in the first place. Psychology teaches us that the way we navigate relationships is shaped by our early experiences. We learn our core beliefs – how we view ourselves, others, and the world — from our environment and primary relationships in our childhood. If basic needs aren't met, our brains adapt in whatever way they can to secure a sense of safety. So, when a child grows up in an unsafe or unstable environment, they will instinctively find ways to cope. Some learn to dissociate, blocking out or ignoring painful experiences. Others become hyper vigilant, constantly scanning for threats to their environment. Additionally, some turn to people-pleasing, while others learn to become invisible, suppressing their own needs entirely. A child will utilize whatever resources they can to survive.

But the very skills that once helped us survive childhood situations become obstacles in adulthood. Where they once worked as tools that kept us safe as children, they now keep us stuck as adults – preventing us from growing and thriving. For a long time, I believed that the past should stay in the past because it couldn't be changed. And while I still believe we can't rewrite history, I now understand that the past shapes who we are in the present. It influences how we think, how we see the world, and ultimately, how we form relationships. If we don't acknowledge and heal those old wounds, we risk sabotaging our own growth — still seeking the safety we never truly had, still longing for the healing we never received.

I have never felt safe. Sure, I have had periods in my life where I felt relatively stable, but they were always fleeting, interrupted by waves of intense sadness and anxiety– at times so heavy it was debilitating. It always seemed like others had a foundation of calm and security that I somehow missed. I have learned as an adult that our ability to cope with stress is shaped in childhood. When we grow up feeling unable to control the stressors in our environment, that sense of helplessness follows us into our adulthood, making it continuously hard to cope with stress effectively. I have struggled with this for most of my life, and it is something I continue to work on.

I remember being maybe six years old, crying in my room, clutching a Polaroid picture of my grandmother, terrified she would die. I sobbed until I couldn't breathe, but no one ever came to comfort me. No one checked to see if I was okay. Often, there was simply no one there. My grandmother lived until I was thirty-one and was rarely sick, so I don't even know where that fear came from. But I do know that fear, sadness, and longing were constants in my childhood.

Even joyful moments felt tainted by an impending sense of loss. I loved Christmas, but every year, I mourned the end of the season. One year, I got the VHS of "Lady and the Tramp" for Christmas. That night, after everyone had gone to bed, I stayed up watching it, looking at our Christmas tree and crying myself to sleep. I must have been around ten. I don't remember a Christmas where I didn't feel that sadness. As an adult, people would laugh at how quickly I "got rid of Christmas." December 26th was a cleaning frenzy for me. I had to get things back to "normal." Otherwise, my mood would drop dangerously low. The emotions I felt as a child – fear, sadness, anxiety – only intensified as I grew older. The duration and times between cycles varied, but the holidays were always a trigger.

Looking back, I can see now that one of the ways I sought safety was through marriage. I believed that having a husband, a lifelong partner, would rescue me from my emotions. That once I had someone to love me unconditionally, I would finally feel safe. But that was never his responsibility, nor something he was capable of doing, even if he tried. When you feel incomplete, you attract others who are also unhealed in some way. I believe that to be true in my case. I drew someone who, like me, had his own struggles.

One of my most profound realizations has been that my issues existed long before my marriage. While my husband and I were unhealthy in a lot of ways, leaving him wouldn't automatically fix me. There was still so much of my past that I needed to confront.

Because the truth is, long before I sought safety in a partner, I had already learned what it meant to live without it. The instability that shaped me didn't begin in my marriage — it began in my childhood, in the shifting dynamics of a family that no longer felt whole. As my parents' relationship unraveled, so did my sense of security. And from that moment on, I would spend years trying to piece it back together, searching for safety in places I was never meant to find it.

***

I don't remember when my mom left. I just remember that she was gone. The few pictures I have from my childhood show the stark difference. When my mother was there, I wore pretty dresses, and my hair was neatly combed. I was laughing in some of the pictures and wore a mischievous smile. There's one photo of my mom and me on Christmas morning, where I am sitting on her lap, holding a stuffed holiday mouse. I think she must have surprised me because we were sitting on my bed, and I looked like I had just woken up. Those times were happy. Then, suddenly, everything changed. There was no warning. No conversation. No goodbye. One day, she was just gone. The mother who had brought me such joy and comfort. Gone.

After that, the pictures of me changed, too. What few there were showed a child who looked disheveled, unkempt, and hollow-eyed. Eventually, the photos stopped altogether.

I was the youngest of seven. Three of us shared the same father. Two of us had the same mother. Only my older brother and I were connected to both. So, when my mother left — taking one daughter from her previous marriage with her, and the other getting married soon after — it was just the five of us left behind with my father, trying to figure things out on our own. Everything about our household changed.

With my mother no longer dressing me, I wore whatever I had lying on the floor in my room – usually my brother's clothes or old hand-me-downs from one of my sisters. My hair was cut short to make it easier to manage. Though I still remember the pain from my hair being yanked into place. The rough brushes through my thick tangles brought tears to my eyes each time. But I never said anything. I didn't complain. By that point, I had already learned to keep quiet to avoid conflict and being a burden. My older sisters, still kids themselves, were now stepping up to take care of my brother and me. Entering their teens, they were beginning to carve out lives of their own while also being expected to hold together the pieces of ours. I'm sure they resented it. Even then, I felt guilt. It was a lonely time for me.

There was no structure. No sense of routine. Just a vague rhythm of survival. I lived in a constant state of uncertainty, unsure of how any given day or night would unfold. My father was trying his best. He worked long hours, doing whatever it took to make ends meet. To this day, I've never met a harder worker than my father. It wasn't until much later that I understood what he was carrying. That he was trying to hold up a household with tired arms and an empty wallet. But when I needed safety and stability the most, all I could feel was that they had disappeared with my mother.

I still saw my mom on some weekends with my brother, and to this day, those weekends at my grandmother's house remain some of the best memories I have. Each time, without fail, we would go to the public library and get books for her to read to us — even long after we could read ourselves. My brother and I would sometimes pick out new books, but we always made sure to grab our familiar favorites.

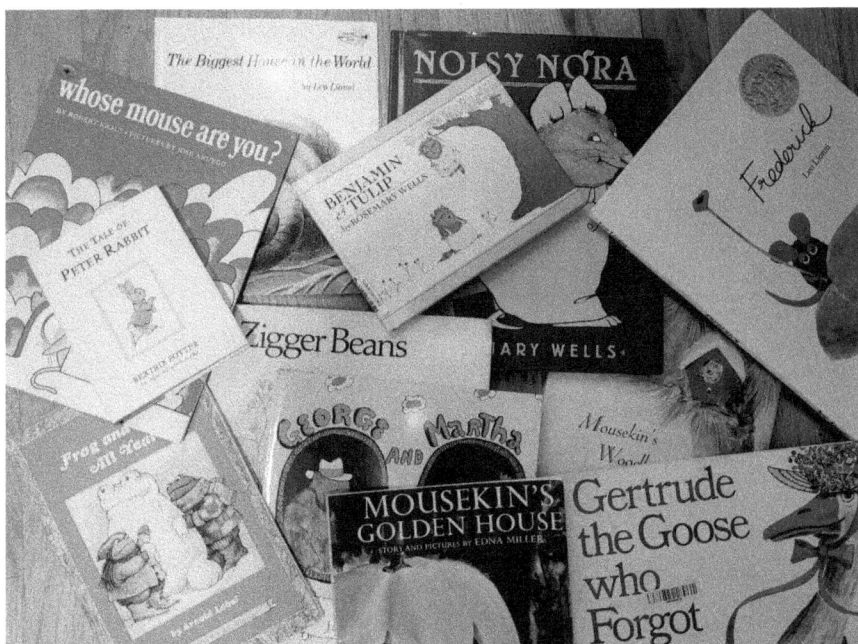

Not long before my marriage ended, I started collecting those same books. Now, a dozen of them sit on a shelf in my closet, small pieces of my childhood tucked away. I hope one day to read them to my grandchildren. Just recently, I found a Frog and Toad T-shirt at a store and bought it for my brother. The memory made me smile. Those books were some of his favorites. I want to continue the memories our mother beautifully created for us.

My mom would take us on walks to the playground at the end of my grandmother's street. In the fall, we would collect beautiful leaves, pine cones, and other interesting foliage, turning them into art projects when we got home. There were no rushed days. Nothing we "had" to do – just the simple joy of showing her our colorful leaves and watching her and my grandmother marvel at our creations. Other times, we would spend hours at the train station, watching the trains go by and waving to the conductor as he tossed candy out of the window for us to catch. Sometimes, we searched for honeysuckles and four-leaf clovers or found entertainment in watching nature shows on TV – back when National Geographic specials were an event, long before cable and on-demand streaming. On warm summer nights, we caught lightning bugs in mason jars (always letting them go before bed), played endless rounds of card games, and watched the stars on my grandmother's front porch. At night, my mother would watch *Tales from the Darkside* and other spooky shows with us in the basement, all of us curled up together in front of the black-and-white TV until we drifted off to sleep.

I knew my mom loved me. Even when we were back at my dad's, she never forgot us. She would call and remind us of all the holiday specials coming up on TV – *The Tale of Peter Cottontail*, *A Charlie Brown Thanksgiving* and Christmas, *Rudolph the Red-Nosed Reindeer*– anything she knew we would like. I can still remember the excitement of turning on the TV to watch our special shows. But when our weekend visits would end, and it was time to leave, a deep fear would settle in me.

Even as a young child, I dreaded stepping out of that safe space, out of that world where, for just a little while, there were no worries, no instability, no uncertainty. At age 47, I have never found a safer place to be. I had a dream a few nights ago that I was back there. When I woke up, I felt a longing that I still don't know how to fill.

Unfortunately, I couldn't live with my mother. Most people assumed it was because she was sick. And it's true – my mother spent much of her time in bed due to chronic back conditions that left her in terrible pain and reliant on medication. But there was a time, after my parents separated, when I did live with her. That's when the first episode of abuse that I can remember began.

At the time, my mother was living with her new husband and his family, and I moved in with them. I don't remember much about the house itself, but my sister recently described it to me as a "party house." There were other adults living there at the time – roommates, I imagine. I was about five years old. My memories of the incidents are clear snapshot images in my brain, while everything before and after remains blurred. I learned through therapy that this is a normal response to trauma.

To put it plainly, I was sexually abused, hated for reasons I could not understand, and living in a constant state of fear over my life. I remember sitting in the tub as a child while they stared back at me with rage-filled eyes. I knew it wouldn't happen in that moment, when people were around, but at some point in the silences of the night, it *would*. I can see my little legs opening up and letting it happen while I detached and went somewhere else in my mind. Now I think, if I had screamed and fought, would that have helped make it stop? I don't know when my screaming stopped. When did I learn quiet resignation?

I remember one incident very clearly. I woke up to someone on top of me, their hands wrapped around my neck. My little hot dog man spun above me, hanging from the ceiling. For some reason, I can still see the vision of my little toy there. Terror flooded my body as I struggled to break free. One moment, I was being strangled. The next, I was on the stairs. I don't know how I got there. I ran down the stairs to find my stepfather watching a war documentary on TV. He was a Vietnam veteran, and his experiences in the war left him with PTSD — something he numbed with alcohol. He was never unkind to me, but I knew to stay away from him when he was drinking, so I hid behind a chair. I was afraid to go back upstairs. Too afraid for him to see me. I don't remember anything after that.

At some point—maybe the next day, maybe later; my timeline is unclear – I crawled in bed with my mother and whispered what had happened. I had to be quiet and sneak into her room because I wasn't supposed to go in there when she was asleep. But she was always sleeping, it seemed. She must have been on a lot of medication that day because she didn't respond to me. I couldn't wake her up no matter how hard I tried. I was defeated after that, knowing I would have to figure out for myself how to stay safe.

Looking back as an adult, I know she heard me. But what could she really do? She had no money of her own, no way of supporting us, no way to take care of us – not with all her medical problems. I needed her to protect me, but she couldn't.

Shortly after I told her what happened, I went back to living with my dad. She did the only thing she could to keep me safe. She gave my father the excuse that I missed my brother and wanted to live with him, keeping me away from the house that brought me danger. It was after that, that our visits with her began to take place at my grandmother's house.

I wonder how bad it must have felt to let me go. I was the last of her children still with her. My brother returned to my dad's before I did — she had to protect him, too.

This was generational trauma. These wounds that my mother carried were passed down. I've heard stories about my great-grandmother losing two of her children due to poverty. Her daughter, my grandmother, grew up during the Great Depression, in a rural, impoverished area of Pennsylvania where resources were scarce and children were expected to be useful. Survival was the only goal, and sometimes love got lost in the scramble. I like to think that with each generation, the suffering lessened. But I can't help but notice the pattern of pain and survival being passed down like heirlooms, wrapped in silence and sacrifice.

I remember my mother as kind. That's the word that lives at the center of her memory: kindness. She adored animals, especially cats. In fact, her charity of choice was the Humane Society. Even in her sickest moments, she made space for the strays. Yet, she too experienced generational trauma passed down from my grandmother and great-grandmother, that would also reach me.

Most of what I know about my mother is pieced together from her, her mother, her last husband, my father, and my oldest sister. Their stories paint a picture of quiet endurance. She was the youngest of two daughters, raised mostly by a single mother. My grandfather was in the Navy and gone for extended periods of time. My grandmother – at least the one I heard about – was a physically and emotionally abusive alcoholic. That's not the version of her I knew; by the time I was born being the youngest of the youngest, she had softened. The stories I heard about her did not align with the way I saw her. But when everyone shares the same memories, the truth becomes undeniable.

I have come to understand that her cruelty likely came from her own brutal upbringing— a result of the stressful impoverished life her mother (my great-grandmother) struggled to raise her in. That is the thing. Pain does not disappear – it evolves, shapeshifts, and seeks new hosts. One story that stands out about my grandmother is how she treated my grandfather when he was dying from cancer. My sister witnessed her scream at him and throw an ashtray at his head while he sat humiliated in his own soiled clothes. Later, I learned that my grandmother perpetrated cruel abuse on my grandfather when he was sick. She would get drunk and stomp on his feet, leaving horrible bruises. He never told anyone, whether it was out of embarrassment, protectiveness, love, guilt, or some other reason I will never know.

I remember my father not caring for my grandmother when I was younger, and not understanding why. After he moved my grandfather—his father-in-law—into our home to protect him from her abuse, my grandfather gave him his old hunting shotgun. He never returned to live with my grandmother. After his death, she asked for the gun back, but my father refused. He later gave that gun to my husband, who has it in a safe for our son Luke, who is sixteen now and hunts fairly regularly with his father. I think my father, my grandfather, and my grandmother would all be satisfied with that arrangement. My father, to this day, has never shared the extent of the abuse, and I am grateful for that. I doubt he ever would have shared anything at all, but I asked when I got older. Sometimes I wish I hadn't. It is still hard to reconcile the grandmother I loved with the woman others feared. The grandmother I knew sang silly songs with me, collected leaves in the fall to create Halloween projects, drove me around looking at Christmas lights, taught me how to play cards, and defended me. She was one of the people I felt safest with.

I guess that's why I feel so strongly about a person's ability to change. I saw it. I lived it.

Surviving the abuse of my grandmother, my mom looked for love, kindness, and companionship wherever she could find it. When I was older, she told me something I'd never expected — that she had been lured into taking nude photographs by an older man as a teenager. This came as we were talking about some of my experiences. It had never occurred to me that my mother might also have had some trauma prior to this conversation. She told me that once she did it the first time, she felt obligated to keep doing it even though it made her feel ashamed and uncomfortable. She hated to hurt anyone's feelings or cause conflict. That kind of people-pleasing made her, like me later, a target for abuse throughout her life. I realized her early trauma shaped her in much the same way mine shaped me.

My mother became pregnant when she was sixteen years old. She was desperate to escape her mother's house, but happiness didn't come with her freedom. Her first child died in her womb at eight months. There were whispers that her abusive husband caused the fall that ended the pregnancy — I don't know for sure. What I do know is that she had to carry that baby, dead inside her, for weeks before her body went into labor. She delivered a baby girl that the hospital never let her hold or grieve. In fact, she was told that was what she deserved for being a young, unwed mother. Her own mother told her that.

Years later, my stepfather bought her a star and named it "Baby Reed" after the child she lost. More than forty years had passed, and yet she wept like it had just happened. My mother generally didn't show a lot of emotion, so it took me by surprise to see her react so strongly. She framed the certificate and kept it near her bedside, always close by. The coordinates of the star are in the form. I have never looked for it, but maybe I will one day. It brings me some comfort to think that if I find that star, I can find where my mom is finally at peace.

She married that man – the father of "Baby Reed'– but he continued to hurt her. He was a cruel and abusive man by everyone's account. He hit her, degraded her. Still, she stayed. That's the cruel loop of generational trauma – it disguises itself as normal. For her, this cycle, which she had experienced since childhood, was familiar, predictable, and in that twisted way, safe. In addition to that, there really was no way out that she could see. Where else could she go? Certainly not home. Move out on her own? She had dropped out of high school and had no skills to support herself or her two kids. This was the seventies – people did not talk about abuse. And when they did, the blame was placed on the women. There was always the hint that you did something to deserve it. I think my mother always believed that to be true.

But the day he hit her daughter was the day something shifted. My oldest sister remembers him slapping her so hard that her glasses flew off and she fell out of her chair. She was six years old at the time. He had crossed a line. My mother could stomach abuse to her, but seeing her child hurt broke something in her. She grabbed a knife and chased him through the house, promising she'd kill him if he ever touched her children again. The marriage ended not long after, and she returned to her parents' home.

She met my father next. He was also divorced, with three children of his own. I do not think you will ever find anyone who has something negative to say about my dad, and that includes his five children and the two children my mother had before their marriage. Now he was no saint by any account, but he was a kind, hardworking, loyal, and honest man. More than anything, he protected her and took care of her children like his own.

My mother's first husband would sometimes come around at his convenience to see his oldest daughter. Other times, he would not show up at all. He continued his sick mind games with my mother, promising to come visit and then never showing up, leaving my sister waiting for hours until she realized he was not coming. At times, he would also choose to pick up my oldest sister and leave the younger one. I guess it was his way of hurting my mother. He knew hurting her kids was more powerful than punching her in the face. When my father witnessed this cruelty, he confronted my mother's ex-husband man to man, making it clear that kind of abuse would no longer be tolerated. Knowing he could not get to my mother anymore, he stopped coming by altogether. Abandoning his daughters, he disappeared.

I'm not sure what led to the breakdown of my parents' marriage. I suspect it had something to do with my mom not knowing how to function in a healthy relationship. Trauma doesn't make room for stability. She may have seen my father as a way to escape her parents' home again, and married more for safety than love. Either way, she eventually chose to leave. As a kid, it hurt. But I am old enough, now, to know that real-life situations are usually more complicated than an outsider realizes. Even from my own experience, I have learned that it was probably a combination of factors that both my mother and my father played a part in.

Her third marriage, to my stepfather, lasted until her death in 2019. He had his demons from the war; she had hers. Somehow, they found solace in each other. Despite her chronic illness and pain, he loved her through it all. I guess she finally found her safe place.

I never stopped needing her, though. Not when I had my first child at 19. Not when I had my daughter at 29. There's a kind of ache that lives in daughters whose mothers are emotionally absent. An ache that doesn't go away. I never blamed her, but I always missed her. Now, she's everywhere in my home. Her spirit lingers in the way I feed stray cats, in the softness I show my own children. It's starting to feel safe here again.

My mother has always been a source of safety and comfort for me. But as I reflect, I recognize patterns and behaviors that weren't normal — things that, woven together with generational trauma, would later shape my sense of security in unsettling ways. Something I remember about both my grandmother and my mother is that they were isolated. Neither of them had friends or hobbies, which didn't seem unusual to me when I was younger. I just assumed that is what happened when you grew up.

My mother, in particular, had chronic pain, so her sleeping during the day and isolating felt like part of her illness as far as I knew. But the older I got, the more I realized that was not the full picture. She also struggled with depression and anxiety, conditions that her medication and self-isolation seemed to numb. I do not want to minimize her pain. She had over fifteen back surgeries, and by the end, the pain was so severe that even high doses of morphine could not manage it. Her quality of life was painfully low. Sometimes I wonder if things might have been different if she had access to non-surgical options earlier, like aqua therapy, stretching, mindfulness, acupuncture, and massage. I will never know.

Even as a child, when people would comment on how much I reminded them of her, it would scare me. I did not want to grow up to be mostly bedridden. Having juvenile rheumatoid arthritis made this fear feel like a prophecy in some ways. I struggled with pain for as long as I can remember. My joints stiffened and ached daily. I took baby aspirin for inflammation and soaked in whirlpool baths for relief. I still remember those bitter, pink chewable pills I took every day.

I suppose I'm lucky I don't remember a time without it. It wasn't like I had a normal childhood and then pain suddenly came — it was always there. I recall some particularly unpleasant camping trips due to this. My father didn't have a lot of money, but he did his best. Every summer, we took a special camping trip to a place called the Wilderness. It was a campground with a small beach, lakes for fishing, a pool, an arcade, and a lot of nature trails. My dad would set up a huge tent for all of us, and we would spend the week exploring. My dad would take us fishing, but mostly my brother and I were left to our own devices. We would swim, ride our bikes, and catch frogs in the lake.

The trips to the Wilderness are mostly good memories for me. It was family time, and I felt free and safe there. The only difficult part of these trips was when it would rain. The tent would leak sometimes, and things would get damp, which significantly aggravated my arthritis. My joints would stiffen to the point where I couldn't sleep. I never told anyone. I just lay there crying silently, stretching and stretching, trying to find relief that never came.

If you've never experienced arthritis pain, the best way I can describe it is that it feels like a stretch you can never quite finish. Your body feels like it *needs* to move in a certain way, but no amount of movement satisfies that feeling. The pain would come and go, but it's the discomfort I remember most. The frustration of never being able to feel okay in my own body.

Somewhere in my teens, the arthritis went into remission. It's stayed that way ever since. But there's always been a quiet fear in the back of my mind — that it might return, or something like it. The fear of being unable to care for myself, bedridden, just like my mother. That fear is probably what created my fierce need to be independent and self-reliant.

Both my mother and my grandmother also had behaviors that would seem "odd" to most people, but growing up around them, they seemed normal. The compulsive cleaning and organizing. The endless lists. Stockpiling canned goods and hygiene products. Hoarding money to the point of self-deprivation. Sleeping during the day and being up at all hours of the night. I remember my grandmother smoking cigarettes and reading books at two or three in the morning. My mother and grandmother both took frequent naps throughout the day and shied away from the outside world. frequently. They feared the public and doctors. They joked about having "OCD" (obsessive-compulsive disorder) as if it were a quirky personality trait, and I accepted it as just that.

It was only later when it appeared in my life that I learned it is much deeper than that. It has always been in my life in one way or another. I had an anxious personality and don't ever remember a time when I didn't exhibit at least some of the behaviors I observed in them. Later in my life, it appeared in a way that was much more frightening– I will go into that later on. OCD and the constellation of symptoms are debilitating. My grandmother managed her anxiety through control and alcoholism. My mother managed hers through passivity, medication, and isolation. As an adult experiencing these symptoms, their behaviors made a lot more sense to me. And I understand them. They did what they could with what they had. For me, there was more awareness, more resources, more support. I can't imagine facing all that without it. It makes me realize how strong they both were.

There were other things I thought were "normal" growing up that absolutely weren't. My older sister used to play a game with my brother and me called "Run, Run, Run, Trip." The whole point was to run across her legs while she tried to trip us — of course, someone always got hurt. It is impossible to run across someone's legs who is trying to trip you and not fall. Usually, it was my brother. He took the brunt of her anger. He ended up in the hospital more than once for what was labeled "roughhousing," but eventually the injuries were serious enough that the hospital suspected abuse.

I was injured once, too. She grabbed one of my arms and legs and spun me around, only to let go abruptly, leaving me to crash into the side of an end table. I was taken to the hospital, where I had to get stitches on the left side of my head near my temple. There is still a faint scar. I recently found out that after my parents separated, my mother took both me and my brother with her. He returned earlier than I did to my dad's house because of my sister's abuse. My mom dropped him off one day, and my dad adjusted to the situation. I assume something similar happened with me when I was not safe with her. My dad just made it work. He took care of us.

In addition to many other things, my older sister had introduced my brother and me to alcohol and cigarettes. Before our teen years, we were allowed to drink and smoke, without objection from our mother. My sister had her own demons. She grew up to struggle with drug addiction and mental illness. When I think about what I experienced as a child, I cannot help but believe she fared far worse. At least I had a father my mom could send me to for safety. My older sister did not have anyone.

My mother used to shoplift, and she taught us how to do it as well. She would take small items, such as earrings or underwear. Sometimes she would direct me to grab something. It felt like a fun game to me. My first shoplift was a pair of gloves from the Ames department store. The gloves didn't fit me, and I didn't even want them. I just took them to be a part of what we were all doing. We would get back into the car and showcase our stolen goods. My grandmother was with us but did not participate. She just laughed and said we shouldn't be doing it. It was all part of life with Mom.

Chapter 2

My Story
(Continued)

Unfortunately for me, there was no safety at my dad's either when I was a child. Like my mom, he did the best he could. He worked extremely hard to provide for five children, with no child support, on a mechanic's salary. And somehow, he always managed to make ends meet. But while he was gone working, I was usually left unsupervised, which made me a prime target for predators.

Maybe this was much more common in the 80s, but at the young ages of six and seven, my brother and I walked to and from school by ourselves. Oftentimes, we were also left at home with no adult supervision. By the time I was six years old, I had met my second abuser. When they asked me if I had ever had sex, I frankly responded "yes." It was just a matter of fact to me at the time. Though, I would regret my answer every day forward. *They* made sure of that.

I was told that if I didn't go along with what they wanted, they would tell everyone about me having sex, with details of all the things I had done — like it was my shame to carry. My fault. That was all it took. I was terrified that my father and others would find out. Worried I would get in trouble. Most of all, I felt shame. And it was a shame I could not escape. This person was in my home, in my community, and in my school. There was no safe place. I did not fight back because I learned with this abuser that it was quicker and easier if I just kept quiet. I would follow them into the closet, where they did the most horrible things, and then go back outside, as if nothing had happened. I literally blocked it out of my mind. It is difficult to describe, because I never forgot any of it. I just ignored it.

As a child, I assumed this kind of thing just happened to some kids. This abuser was not just physically abusive, but psychologically cruel as well. They seemed to enjoy frightening me and making me do perverse acts just to see the fear and disgust on my face. Some of the abuse happened in my own home, in my own room, just down the hall from my siblings. When this person would come into my room, I had two options: "truth or dare" or "would you rather" - both horrible. Though Truth or Dare was worse. Truth would require me to admit things out loud about myself that they knew to be true, but caused me to feel shame and humiliation. It goes without saying, the dare was just as bad.

Sometimes, the abuse would happen at their house. I remember one thing this person enjoyed doing was squeezing my hand very tightly to force my knuckles together. The juvenile rheumatoid arthritis I had as a child made my joints, especially in my hands and feet, very sensitive and stiff. So, when my hand was squeezed, the pain was so horrible it felt like it was going to break. I remember acting like it didn't hurt, even though there would be tears in my eyes. I never let myself fully cry. If I cried, it would be acknowledging some kind of terrible truth that I did not want to believe. In my young mind, I was convinced that all of these events, while horrible, were just a part of being a kid. I guess I knew that not everyone experienced these things, but I thought it was simply how life was for me. To cry would mean I had to accept that something was terribly wrong and distorted.

Trying to describe and rationalize what my young mind believed is difficult, but I still understand her. When I remember the events, it is as if I am an observer of the abuse. I can see myself from above. There are many gaps in my memory from these experiences, and I am grateful for that. In my young mind, I was disgusting, and I never even thought about saying anything to anyone because I believed that I deserved it. I remember constantly being ashamed of this secret, and never being able to make that feeling go away. The abuse — and the shame it brought with it — continued until we moved again. I was nine by then.

Although I was physically safe when we moved — no longer experiencing the abuse — I don't remember *feeling* safe. I longed for mutual connection with people, but did not know how to get it, or even accept it when it came. This made me a walking contradiction. On one hand, I desperately feared abandonment. I remember, for example, crying at night, fearing my grandmother was going to die, even when she was perfectly healthy. Or how empty I felt when my older siblings got married and moved out, leaving just my brother and me. On the other hand, though, I had trouble letting people in. My father remarried, and his wife tried to form a connection with me, but by that time, I was scared to trust anyone else. Fear culminated with rage. I used it against myself as a teenager and anyone else who got a little too close. At the time, it felt like I was the only one affected. My brother seemed relatively stable. I realized only recently, however, that he did not escape our childhood unscathed either. And in his adulthood, as he shared, he also struggled to emotionally connect with people, which devastated most of his relationships. Out of respect for his privacy, that's all I will share.

When I was twelve years old, I rode my bike through my usual trail to get to my best friend Joanna's house. Out of nowhere, a naked man came out of the woods and blocked my path. He looked at me and asked if I knew what his private part was. "Yes," I said. I didn't scream or run, I just stayed there looking at him, and finally asked if I could leave.

Amazingly, he simply said yes and walked back into the woods. I rode my bike to my friend's house and told her what happened. It didn't really occur to me that this was a "big deal." I never expected it to become an issue, but her mother called the police, and my father was notified. I was able to pick him out of a lineup of pictures the police showed me, and he confessed. I learned that he had previously "flashed" some kids at a bus stop. It was really eye-opening to see the books of Polaroid pictures the police had with all of these men out on the street who were known to be predators. Something I remember from this experience was thinking, "but he didn't even do anything". To me, this was not something I considered traumatic. I still don't. I think that's why I wanted to include it here. It shows that on some level, I was kind of numb to this type of thing.

Another instance that stands out happened to me in ninth grade. I was in the Frost school at the time, an alternative school for teens with behavioral and/or emotional issues. I remember falling asleep on the school bus and a boy touching me between my legs. Although I woke up instantly, I pretended to stay asleep. This time, the harassment didn't come from an authority figure or even someone older or bigger. He was just some kid in my class. And still, I didn't say anything. Didn't move. Didn't stop him. I just froze. To this day, I struggle with the fact that I *let* him touch me. Logically, I understand that freezing is a trauma response, but knowing that somehow doesn't absolve me of the shame I still feel. I continue to fight hard to challenge this way of thinking. But at the time, instances like these made these experiences feel routine — inevitable.

In addition to the sexual harassment and abuse, I struggled socially. In middle school, I was bussed to a predominantly Black school as part of the "TAG" program – Talented and Gifted. I didn't understand it at the time, but now it's clear why the other kids resented me. White kids from the suburbs were brought into their school and placed in special classes for "smart kids," so that they were largely excluded from. I had no idea that I was a pawn in some messed-up, racist policy, but being at that school was awful for me.

Those kids hated me. I was not just white — I was pale, blond, skinny, unathletic, and not yet developed. They called me all kinds of names, but mostly "ghost". I remember feeling painfully self-conscious about my body, which was flat-chested and immature compared to the other girls. I also started hating my complexion and found ways to hide my skin whenever I could. Before going to that school, I barely thought about it unless I had sunburn.

The kids would grab my hair, make fun of the way I dressed, and find something to pick on in almost everything I did. I hated them too — but more than anything, I just wanted to be like them. I envied the way their mothers did their hair in intricate designs. Same with the clothes they wore, and the closeness so many of them seemed to share.

By the time I was a teenager, all that pain turned into fear and rage, and it started coming out in a number of ways — alcohol and drug use, shoplifting, acting out sexually, and self-harm. In ninth grade, I stopped going to school altogether. The panic I felt every day was intolerable. I couldn't even explain what I was afraid of — and honestly, I still can't. But it was real. Palpable. I would do anything to avoid that bus. I'd hide in my closet all day or disappear into the woods near the church across the street, even when it was freezing. Anything was better than going back to that place. There wasn't one major incident that triggered it. I dealt with the usual school bullies, but nothing worse than what other kids went through. I was actually a good student — smart, capable — but I always felt like I didn't belong. That feeling didn't come from the other kids. It came from *me*, so there was no escaping it.

At this point, my father was very concerned about me and, frankly, didn't know what to do. This was new territory for him. The firm discipline that worked with his four previous children would not work with me. My mom's approach was the opposite. As a teenager, her parenting became very permissive. She allowed me to smoke and drink, and even knew that I had taken some of her prescription medication. She could not stand to see me in pain, so if I said I needed something, she gave it to me. What I really craved was her love, but it was inconsistent. She couldn't always be there. There was no solution to my pain that I could see.

My first psychiatric hospitalization happened when I was fifteen years old after a suicide attempt by overdose. I was taken to the Psychiatric Institute of Montgomery County. I don't remember much about the hospital other than tests and being angry. I didn't really want to die; I just didn't want to feel that way anymore. But nothing changed. None of the medications they tried improved my mood, and I was not interested in trusting a therapist. I was hospitalized two more times as a teenager for similar reasons. My father kept my discharge papers in his room. When I found them, there were five different diagnoses listed: manic depression (bipolar), depression, anxiety, panic disorder, and substance abuse disorder. I don't believe PTSD was ever listed on any of the discharge diagnoses.

In many ways, my teenage years were more difficult than my childhood. At least in my childhood, I knew who the boogeyman was. There was a clear source of fear and, however dysfunctional, a way to survive. Even if it meant dissociating from the abuse, I had an escape. But as a teen, the fear felt everywhere and nowhere at the same time. I couldn't point to it. It just felt unsafe in my own skin. I tried to run from it — with alcohol, drugs, sex, stealing, and self-harm. But the feeling always returned. All I could do was keep running to avoid it.

As my behaviors became riskier and more unpredictable, I lost contact with my friends from school. I attached myself to the "bad kids," never developing any real friendships. Mostly, I drank a lot of alcohol and used acid and marijuana. Much of that time is a blur. I was trying to escape the heavy, hollow feeling inside me — that constant undercurrent of fear, loneliness, and disconnection. Well-meaning therapists tried to help, but by the time they stepped in, it felt like the damage had already been done.

In my sophomore year of high school, I was placed in a school for students with behavioral problems. They tried to offer me homeschooling as well, but none of the interventions were successful because by that time, I had tasted the freedom that substances, acting out, and avoidance could bring. It wasn't real freedom, but it gave me a sense of control — the only control I felt I had. The professionals had no answers that made me feel better.

Despite everything, academics were never an issue. Even with all the chaos and missed school days, I excelled in my courses. But then, at sixteen, I was arrested for stealing polo shirts from Nordstrom at the Annapolis Mall. My mother bailed me out, and the only consequence was being banned from the store. Shortly after, I dropped out of school. From the outside, it must have looked like I was spiraling. And maybe I was. But deep down, I didn't want to ruin my life — I just didn't know how to save it. What I wanted was safety, security, and stability. I just didn't know how to find it. Looking back now, I know my acting out was a cry for help.

Fortunately, a falling out with a peer who was involved in a local crime ultimately became a turning point for me. It made it necessary for me to leave the county and cut ties with the crowd I'd been running with. It didn't bother me. I wasn't close with anyone anyway. At almost eighteen, I moved in with my oldest sister. She provided the structure and stability I needed, and for the first time in a long while, I started making real changes in my life. I earned my GED and enrolled in college. I even got a job at a gas station and met my first real boyfriend. That constant need for safety never left me, though, and soon after we started dating, I became pregnant. It wasn't planned, but I wasn't using protection either. On some level, I think that I wanted a baby — someone who I would have forever. I know it sounds selfish and immature. It wasn't like it was a conscious plan or anything, but our choices usually come from somewhere.

From the moment I found out I was pregnant, everything changed. I stopped using drugs and alcohol. I took on two jobs to prepare financially, and I stayed in school because I wanted a career — a way to take care of this baby. I now had a purpose. And for a while, the anxiety and instability faded. Of course, like many things in life, that peace was temporary. My son's father and I did not work out, and he proved incapable of being the parent our son needed, so I stepped into the role on my own. I was a teenage single parent, doing the very best I could with limited resources — but I loved my son deeply and never wavered in providing for him.

Thankfully, I had some help along the way. One of the biggest supporters was a family I worked for as a Nanny. This was a full-time job that allowed me to bring my son. I got paid in cash and didn't have to worry about daycare. This arrangement helped me complete my Associate's degree and land an entry-level job in my field by the time my son entered kindergarten. I was even able to afford my own townhome. I also kept up with my education. I took classes for over eight years, eventually earning my Bachelor's degree, and later went on to pursue a Master's degree. It was a slow process, but my strengths were patience, focus, and being goal-oriented. I never wanted to have to depend on someone to take care of me financially. If I ever ended up alone, I wanted to be able to provide for myself.

From the outside, I appeared completely transformed from my rebellious teenage years. I had a career and my own home as a single mom in my mid-20s. But if I could talk to that young woman now, I'd tell her that even though things looked different, I was still carrying so much inside. I was still lonely. Still afraid. I had little confidence in myself and still searched for that missing piece. On top of that, I carried a lot of the anxious, compulsive patterns I'd inherited from my mother and grandmother. I couldn't relax. I was often isolated — even when I wasn't physically alone. My problems were still mine.

I let It Grow

Chapter 3

My Husband's Story

Some people who experience trauma become perpetrators of the same type of trauma. I became an empath — a person deeply attuned to the feelings and needs of others. I've always had, and still have, an innate desire to heal the broken, to love the unloved, and bring happiness to those around me. It's a quality that can make someone a compassionate partner, a loyal friend, a nurturing mother, and a dedicated worker. But without boundaries and self-awareness, it can also lead to self-sacrifice and destruction at the hands of those who manipulate and misuse that kindness.

Empaths are often people pleasers who place the needs and desires of others above their own. Because we worry that people will not love us, we try to make them *need* us. But here's the thing —self-sacrifice sometimes comes with hidden expectations. There's often an unspoken hope that others will give back in the same way. And when they don't, resentment starts to build. People pleasers usually struggle to express their needs, believing others should intuitively *und*erstand, just as we're attuned to everyone else. This disconnect leaves us with unmet emotional needs and a persistent sense of being taken advantage of or overlooked.

Alongside that, I developed an anxious-avoidant attachment style in my relationships — a mix of craving deep emotional intimacy while simultaneously feeling overwhelmed and fearful of it. It's a push-pull dynamic that might seem contradictory but is a common response to trauma. And it's incredibly confusing — not just for me, but for the person I'm with. There were days when I craved intimacy and affection. Other days, I needed total isolation. Even small emotional asks or physical affection from my partner felt like suffocation, and I'd get irritated or angry for reasons I couldn't always explain. I remember talking to a friend of mine before my marriage. I was pulling into my driveway, and my then-fiancé, who had recently moved in, was already home. I was frustrated by his presence because I had been looking forward to some time alone. She reminded me: "You're marrying this guy. He's always going to be there."

My husband didn't reveal any signs of having an unhealthy or traumatic childhood, at least not early in our marriage. It wasn't until much later on that he shared that with me, and even then, it was unintentional. More matter of fact. He hadn't recognized that what he experienced was unhealthy. To him, it was just the way things were.

From the outside, his family looked like the picture of stability. His parents had been together since shortly after they graduated from high school. He had two brothers who appeared successful by most standards, and a large extended family with no divorces or visible signs of dysfunction. He attended private school, and the whole family went to church every Sunday. He and his brothers were altar servers, their mom volunteered at school, and their dad was a Eucharistic minister who also coached their Little League teams. They celebrated birthdays and holidays together, and everyone seemed to get along.

But there's no such thing as a perfect family. Even the ones that look pristine on the outside can carry hidden wounds. I don't say this to be critical or to cast blame. I say it to offer context — just as my past shaped me, I wanted to understand how his shaped him.

Eventually, I started having conversations with my sisters-in-law, and I realized our stories overlapped. All three brothers had patterns of behavior that were hard to ignore: a lack of empathy, emotional distance, and trouble managing anger. Stonewalling and silent treatment were common tactics. We found ourselves trying to piece it all together — what had happened in that household to leave such a mark on each of them?

By then, we'd started to notice certain dynamics within the family that were concerning — things they considered normal, but to us felt troubling. My husband shared that, growing up, his older brother, six years his senior, had been allowed to fight him. I don't mean your typical sibling roughhousing. I mean actual physical fights. At just seven years old, he was regularly beaten by a thirteen-year-old. When they argued, they were told to "take it outside," and with such a gap in age and strength, his older brother was never the one to lose. My husband learned to avoid him as much as possible, but in a small house, there was only so much space to retreat. His brother thrived on asserting dominance, and the physical threats were constant. It got to the point where my husband would hold off on going to the bathroom just to avoid leaving his room and risking a confrontation.

One of my first interactions with his brother involved him ridiculing my son, and my reaction was seen as "over the top." He masked cruelty as a joke. To this day, my husband doesn't see it as abusive. We agreed to disagree on that. Growing up in his family, emotions — especially the so-called "weak" ones like sadness and fear — were not allowed. He learned early on to compartmentalize. Showing vulnerability was a risk. Both of his parents were emotionally distant, and love was conditional. You earned approval through compliance and achievement.

His older brother was the classic straight-A student, the type who could memorize and regurgitate information to ace a test. My husband was not that kind of student. He did well, but not exceptionally, like his brother, and he was constantly reminded of it. His intelligence manifested in different ways – he was quick, creative, and resourceful. Leave him with anything, and he could figure it out. He was a lot like his mother in that regard, but that intelligence wasn't celebrated. Though if you ask me, that's the kind that really matters.

Instead, he grew up thinking that he was deficient somehow — like something in him needed to be "fixed." He recalls being put on medication to help him with school, but the side effects became too much. No one asked what he needed; they just tried to make him fit the mold. Feelings simply were not discussed. He has no memory of affection from his parents — no "I love you," no hugs. And even now, I can see his deep longing for love and approval from his father.

The relationship between his parents was what you might call "old school." He worked and provided financially, and she took care of the house and kids. There was a dynamic in their marriage where he was the one in charge. Rarely did I see him compliment or show any outward expression of affection. The boys picked up on that dynamic. All three of them mirrored that same emotional detachment when interacting with their mother.

For her part, she grew resentful and bitter. She never voiced her needs, but would become angry when those needs weren't met, leaving everyone around her guessing. Her communication style was passive-aggressive and difficult to navigate. I never knew where I stood with her. If she was upset, I'd often find out through someone else in the family, never from her directly. As grandparents, it was frustrating to witness the constant comparisons between the grandchildren and how they seemed to compete for affection. It's a long-running family joke that she keeps a mental list of favorites. And while she laughs it off and insists that's not true, we could all recite that list in perfect order.

Amidst this complicated family dynamic, my husband recalls a time when he felt his father was proud of him. By his early twenties, after a lifetime of being bullied by his older brother, he had finally grown strong enough to fight back. An altercation broke out between them, and this time, he refused to back down. He stood his ground and left his brother with two black eyes. That was the last time they fought. Like most bullies who pick on younger, weaker targets, once they are no longer able to dominate, the behavior tends to stop. That evening at dinner, his father cracked a smile when he found out. That smile, subtle as it was, meant everything to my husband. It was the closest thing to approval he could remember. As for his brother, he grew older and matured, just like the rest of us. He's not the villain in this story. There is no villain. At one point or another, we all play the villain in someone else's story.

My husband developed an avoidant attachment style as a way to cope with his fear of rejection and deep-seated feelings of inadequacy. Of course, that's my interpretation of his behavior, not an official diagnosis or even something he would necessarily agree with. But in our marriage, it showed up as a lack of empathy, a fear of emotional vulnerability, and extreme defensiveness — especially when he felt criticized, even slightly. With my own insecure attachments, I was drawn to his emotional distance. I had the same fear of emotional intimacy. The problem was that I also deeply craved the very thing I feared, and not getting that need met would be a trigger for the emotional unraveling I experienced in my early forties. The crisis that landed me back in the hospital, wondering how the cycle from my teenage years had come back again, almost thirty years later.

Sharing these parts of our childhood is not an attempt to deflect accountability for our adult behaviors and decisions. I believe that most people, especially parents, do the best they can with what they know and the resources available to them. I shared what I knew about my mother's experience, which will undoubtedly invite the reader to feel compassion for her. However, I couldn't do the same for either of my husband's parents, simply because I don't know their story. Still, I believe, like all of us, they have one — one that might explain the patterns, the emotional distance, and the choices they made. My husband once shared with me that he believes his parents did what they thought was right — raising boys to be strong in an unkind world. To them, building a strong work ethic, independence, and self-sufficiency was the priority. To them, emotional resilience meant hiding feelings and pushing through.

This isn't about blame and judgment. It's about understanding. About making sense of how things got to be the way they were and choosing to rewrite that story moving forward. Because I don't believe healing can happen without accountability. Looking back helps you make sense of what you don't realize when you're in the middle of it.

Chapter 4

The Marriage

Of course, it started out as a thrilling romance between my husband and me. Isn't that how it is for most of us? He was everything I had ever wanted in a man — handsome, kind, funny, and smart. He had a good job, was financially secure, and desired a long-term, committed relationship. He was dependable — safe. I clung onto that. In those early days, I only saw the good in him.

We were drawn to each other for many of the same reasons any other couple is — physical attraction, shared interests, and simply enjoying each other's company. But what made our connection different was that we both had insecure attachment styles that neither of us realized at the time. His upbringing with his emotionally unavailable parents made him **avoidant**, unable to express emotional intimacy in his relationships. My inconsistent childhood environments, on the other hand, left me **disorganized** (both anxious and avoidant), in which I experienced a mix of craving intimacy and similarly avoiding it. This created a volatile dynamic in our relationship, where we *seemed* to have what the other wanted, but failed to satisfy each other's deeper needs.

The "love bombing" phase at the beginning of the relationship made things seem bright and promising. This is typical for avoidant attachers; they create a seemingly close connection early on that they are unable to maintain due to their fear of real intimacy. In that initial stage, he made me feel loved and valued in a way I never had before. He told me everything I wanted to hear: I was beautiful, smart, talented, strong, and *different* from his other exes. I was special. He furnished my entire home with new furniture and took me places I had never been before. Those first six months were magical. I truly believed he was my soulmate, that I had finally found the one person who would love me forever. After each day, we would talk on the phone for hours or send long emails. And in those moments, I could tell him things I had never shared with anyone. He made me feel safe — a feeling I had searched for since childhood. I would do anything to keep that. So, I quickly attached and became fiercely loyal. I idolized him.

Obviously, this did not last. Eventually, his avoidance came out, and I no longer felt the safety I once depended on him for. Although we both shared a fear of intimacy, I also had the side of me that craved it. So, the mutual expectation of not being emotionally available did not always work for me. I wanted more. And my inconsistency confused him. We proved not to be what each other needed. This is not to say that our marriage was all bad. It wasn't even mostly bad, despite what you will read. But when it was bad, it was *awful*. Still, there was comfort in the stability of his presence. There was companionship. We had some truly wonderful times. In fact, some of my best memories are with him — and, admittedly, some of my worst.

While I was pregnant with my daughter, I was working full-time and going to school while he built our home. Every evening after work and all weekend long, he was there, turning the dream we had sketched out on paper into reality. Both of us were incredibly hard workers — driven, and goal-oriented. We had that in common. We also shared a Christian faith, and it was important to us that we raise our children in that tradition.

I still remember sitting in our home after it was built, marveling that something so beautiful was ours — and that *he* had made it happen. We celebrated all our milestones together — graduations, promotions, and anniversaries. With the kids, we would wake up at 4 AM together each Christmas morning to work "Santa's" magic under the tree. And when Easter rolled around, it was a team effort to find the best hiding spots for the eggs. There were really amazing moments.

Even before we married, when he worked out of state, I would visit him for long weekends. It would be just the two of us, dreaming and planning our future together. Now, it was here. And it was amazing, at least for a moment.

Love and marriage aren't about the magical first few years, though. That initial phase, where both people put their best selves forward, eventually comes to an end. He began to see that I had flaws, and I realized he couldn't fix everything that was broken in me. This is the natural progression of any relationship, not unique to just ours. The idealization phase ends for everyone. What made our marriage particularly challenging was our inability to deal with the conflict once it arose.

The biggest struggle was communication. My husband was very sensitive to criticism, so any mention of an issue felt like a personal attack and made him extremely defensive. Looking back, it makes sense — his family dynamic had conditioned him to expect scrutiny rather than celebration. But his sensitivity placed me back into a familiar role of walking on eggshells to avoid conflict. Just like in my father's house growing up, I learned to tolerate the intolerable in silence, just to keep the peace. Things that should have been unacceptable became acceptable if it meant avoiding an argument.

I had become accustomed to agreeing with him on pretty much everything, unless I had a very strong opinion —

and was prepared to deal with the inevitable conflict, which I detested. When we argued, he would simply shut down, giving me the silent treatment and withholding emotional support and affection. This behavior started relatively early in our relationship and was extremely effective because of my fear of abandonment and rejection. I would do almost anything to avoid it. It was more important for me not to upset him than it was not to upset myself. I found myself constantly anticipating what might make him unhappy and trying to fix it before it became a problem.

Early in our marriage counseling, we proudly remarked that we "never argued." The therapist gently explained that this was actually a sign of an unhealthy relationship. Problems and disagreements arise in every marriage. When they do, you have two choices: you can deal with them or let them grow. We let them grow.

I wasn't innocent in this dynamic. I mirrored unhealthy patterns too — sometimes being extremely affectionate, then shutting down emotionally when he got too close or challenged me in ways I wasn't ready to face. Once I knew his vulnerabilities, I sometimes weaponized them, using emotional distance to push him away — until I craved that connection again. We hurt each other.

One memory I will never forget is my labor with our daughter in 2007. She was a beautiful, perfect eight-pound baby, though the birthing experience wasn't quite so wonderful. After a difficult experience with my son's birth, we decided on a birthing center rather than a hospital. We carefully planned for a natural birth and non-medicinal interventions for pain. But as my labor progressed and the pain became overwhelming, I decided I needed something for the pain — a decision that was not part of our plan. I knew my husband would disapprove.

After I was given a shot of morphine, he left the room, leaving me in labor alone.

It triggered my deepest fears of abandonment on what should have been one of the most wonderful and special days of our lives. I remember it vividly — kind of like the snapshots of my childhood traumas. I can still see myself, alone in that room, in so much pain, terrified that I had upset him, and desperately wanting him to come back. I could hear him in the other room with the midwife laughing and joking about something. He thought the medication would stop the sharp pain of the contractions, or that I would fall asleep, but if you've ever given birth, you know that doesn't happen. It barely dulled the pain.

He came back only when I was delivering her. He was the first to touch our daughter, beaming while he cut the umbilical cord, as if nothing was wrong at all. He was a happy, glowing father. I, on the other hand, fell into postpartum depression after her birth. A few days after we came home, I tried to talk to him about what had happened. He told me I had yelled at him during labor, that I told him to leave the room. In his mind, the matter was settled. But for me, it was just the beginning. I didn't press it. I didn't explain how I felt or what I needed. Like so many things between us, I let it grow. When I talked to a good friend of mine about it, she sounded horrified, so much so that I didn't even tell her the whole story. I knew what she would say, what she would think, and I wasn't prepared to hear it. I kept a lot of secrets that way. It became my shame, because really, who just lets something like that go?

In our marriage, my husband exhibited persistent patterns of behavior, such as the silent treatment and withholding affection, when he was angry. I desperately tried to gain his affection and approval, even if it meant suppressing my own needs. I felt emotionally afraid and uncertain in my own home, in my own skin. I didn't even know my own likes and preferences, because everything I did was to please someone else. I had built a life that fit the narrative from my childhood. I needed to be of service. I needed people to need me, because without that, I didn't feel worthy of love. I had no boundaries. I didn't know what my needs were, much less how to articulate them to anyone else.

On the rare occasion when I told him he hurt my feelings or suggested that he had done something wrong, he became defensive. He would never apologize. Instead, he suggested I was taking things the wrong way, that I was too sensitive, or even denied what happened altogether. He would point to my history of mental health issues and trauma, implying that I was hyper-aware and overly sensitive. Over time, I stopped trusting my own feelings and started relying on him — and others — to tell me how I should feel.

He was unable to support me emotionally or show empathy when I experienced sadness or difficulty. Early in our marriage, both of us were comfortable with this arrangement. We didn't share our difficult feelings or troubles. We silently agreed to a "no-conflict" policy. While I always wanted more, I was terrified that if I asked for it, I would be rejected, so I never did. I accepted what he was able to offer, and I offered the same.

The push and pull I described in my attachment style led me to marry someone who would inevitably reject my emotional needs. I was too afraid to seek intimacy out in a partner because it was threatening, so I ended up with someone unable to provide it. Years into our marriage, I realized I needed more. I tried to confide in him about my feelings, especially as my mental health started to deteriorate. But the only way I can describe it is that he had a switch. When things became too heightened for him, he could simply turn it all off. I envied that ability. When I pulled away out of fear, I always felt the desperate longing for connection. It was almost as if I could feel enough for both of us.

I think I could have lived that way — with some semblance of happiness — forever if it weren't for the children. I had brought my son into the marriage, and my husband was unable to connect with him. He made some efforts to involve him in activities he enjoyed, including different sports, racing, and hunting, but my son was not an outdoorsman. He was more artistic and creative. Neither was particularly enthusiastic about the other. I would describe their relationship as apathetic roommates. They mostly ignored each other.

There were times when my husband attempted to discipline my son, but I felt it wasn't balanced by affection and love, so I didn't allow it. I explained away my son's behavior, and I was very guarded and protective of their interactions. In truth, I had picked up some of my mother's parenting behaviors. I was overly permissive, trying to mow down any and all obstacles my son might face — partly to avoid the uncomfortable emotions that come with life's inevitable difficulties. I wanted everything to be "okay" all the time and felt deeply uneasy with conflict and the normal ups and downs of life. My husband and I were very much alike in that way: sweep it under the rug and keep it moving. We used different means to achieve the same end.

One of the biggest issues in our marriage arose from our differing parenting styles, particularly regarding our daughter. There was no apathetic roommate situation between my husband and our daughter. She was a "Daddy's girl" from the beginning and lived off his approval and affection. She was smart, beautiful, kind, funny, and athletic. It's the last trait that changed everything. *Athletic*. She was naturally gifted, and her talent was evident from an early age. She could run with ease and throw a ball better than most boys. She had inherited her father's spatial awareness and agility. Softball became the love of her life at age seven, when she was invited to play on a travel team with girls much older than her.

Looking back, I wish we had declined that offer. Yes, she was talented enough. But she wasn't mature enough — and neither her father nor I fully understood what we were getting into with the world of travel sports. At first, we all enjoyed the attention and praise she received from it, at first. She loved the special attention, especially from her father. It started out innocently enough. She joined a local team and traveled to nearby tournaments. It was fun for her and for us. But at some point, the sport stopped being about fun and started being about "college prep." It started when her father began coaching.

You always want the trauma to stop with you, but you never quite know how to make that happen. My daughter was just as much of a people pleaser as I was. The person she most wanted to make happy was her father. She pushed through injuries and put a smile on her face long after she stopped enjoying the sport. Still, somehow it never felt like what she did was enough. Off-season conditioning, private coaching, national teams — it became more like a full-time job than a hobby. It was all-consuming. There was no time for other interests, no space for friendships. And she was terrified to tell him she didn't want to do it anymore.

I could see it happening. But I wasn't much help. I am ashamed to say it now, but I didn't want the conflict. I was too busy trying to make the problems disappear without actually dealing with them. Any time he was unkind, I would step in — not to confront him, but to soften the blow, to do something nice, to patch it over. But I never stopped it.

Less than two years after our daughter was born, we had a son. He wasn't as much of a people pleaser, but he had his own way of surviving the toxicity in our home: he did everything right. Not poorly, not too great, just good enough to avoid notice and stay off the radar as much as possible.

I didn't like the way my husband — and the men in his family — treated people, especially their children. There was a pattern: "Do what I say," with no room for love, compassion, emotions, or healthy conflict. Looking back, I realize that there were numerous opportunities for me to step in, speak up, and create change. But out of fear, I never did. Instead, I avoided. I separated. I became quietly angry over the things I was too afraid to name out loud.

The kids and I went on vacations with my sister or my friends to visit family. My husband wasn't invited on these trips. I thought I was creating space for the kids and myself, but all I was really doing was widening the divide. It alienated him even more, bred more animosity and resentment. He was hurt, but he didn't know how to name that hurt or express it. And in his family, that was just the way things were: you accepted it, or you coped in destructive ways. Hindsight is 20/20. You don't get second chances in life. But if I could make one change, it would be this: I would have spoken up. I would have demanded a change. I would have done something useful. At that time, in that place, I could have intervened and made a difference for my children, my husband, my marriage, and myself. But I didn't. I couldn't. I tell myself that I did the best I could with what I knew and the resources I had at that time — and that's true. But it doesn't make it right. My fear made it impossible for me to act.

I told my therapist once that I hated to see my kids suffer. She said, "Maybe you don't like to see yourself suffer." It was the first time I considered that my actions weren't purely benevolent. I could talk endlessly about the importance of letting kids experience natural consequences, about building resilience, but in practice, I often denied them that opportunity because I couldn't tolerate my own discomfort. It wasn't about protecting them from pain. It was about protecting myself from feeling helpless. It was something my husband had often tried to tell me, but I had angrily defended my parenting. I was guilty of being defensive, guilty of emotionally distancing myself when he brought up issues I wasn't ready to face.

I wish that knowing solved everything. The more I learned, the more everything made sense. But it didn't magically make change easier. All the reasons I built those patterns were still there, deeply rooted. Behavior that is rewarded is repeated, after all. I had to figure out: what were the rewards for my behaviors? What did they give me? And did I really want to change, or did I just want the consequences of my behaviors to change?

If I truly wanted change, I had to figure out how to get those needs met in healthier ways. I had to face what I had allowed to grow for eighteen years in my marriage, and for almost my whole life before that.

Chapter 5

Beyond 'Happily Ever After'

In 2017, I started therapy again. The anxiety and depression I had struggled with in childhood and adolescence never truly went away. Maybe I'd just been so busy being a mother and working that I was able to keep it on "simmer" for a while. But at forty years old, it began to reawaken — the same old, familiar feelings I dreaded. That year marked the beginning of the most painful period of my life, something I'm still trying to recover from today.

I felt unsafe again. I thought marriage, children, a steady job, and financial stability — earning a master's degree and holding a comfortable position with the State — would bring me security. I was wrong. On the outside, everything looked fine. No apparent issues, no visible concerns. Looking back now, I see so many moments where change was possible, though I didn't have the wisdom then that I have now. At that time, I didn't know what to do with the overwhelming emotions I was experiencing. My first instinct was to ignore them and shove them down. Unsurprisingly, that didn't work.

I started therapy, but it wasn't helpful. The focus was mainly on managing anxiety with breathing techniques, relaxation, mindfulness, and distraction. We never addressed the root cause, so the anxiety just kept getting worse. I started having terrifying panic attacks in the early morning. I would wake from a dead sleep with my heart racing, nauseous, cold, disoriented, and with an overwhelming fear...of nothing? To make matters worse, I hid these symptoms from everyone, including my husband. I was ashamed. Afraid he would think I was "crazy" and leave me. The panic would fade as the day went on, but over time, it became more and more difficult to manage on my own. Therapy wasn't effective, so I stopped going.

Sadly, I existed like that for nearly a year. I wasn't really present in anything I was doing; I was just trying to survive. One of the most heartbreaking parts of all this is the time I lost with my children. I wasn't truly there for so much of their childhood. I tried to work through it by journaling, exercising, and eventually returning to therapy. I even tried neurofeedback and psychiatric medications. But despite these efforts, I continued to decline. I eventually opened up to my husband, but even then, I gave him the "G-rated" version of what I was really experiencing. By the time I fully admitted how bad things had gotten, the anxiety and panic had evolved into a deep depression I couldn't control, no matter how hard I tried.

I cried constantly. I locked myself in my room to hide from the kids, and wore sunglasses when I had to take them out to the bus stop. I couldn't eat and lost a significant amount of weight. I couldn't sleep. I felt hopeless, unseen, and burdensome. I would even leave work early just to sit in my car and cry. I had convinced myself that no one cared about me and that the world would be better if I were gone. One day, I came across an Instagram reel that said, "There are some people alive today only because their kids are." That summed up my experience perfectly.

In a journal from that time, I wrote:

"I wish I didn't have the responsibility of my kids because it would be so much easier to just get rid of my pain."

"That's how I think today, anyway. But how much longer will that thought be enough?"

"Is it better to have a sick mom or a dead mom? Does it even matter if I don't function either way?"

"Maybe Darryl would be better off with a new wife who — one who can be a good mom."

Here is an excerpt from a journal I wrote during that same timeframe:

6/6/18

I was suicidal again this morning.

I sat in the tub and stared at the razor.

The thought of the blade slicing the veins in my wrist

I didn't think much about the pain — maybe a burning, stinging throb.

No, I wondered if the blood would carry away the dark feelings.

I imagined a calm overtaking my body and mind, and finally being free.

Instead, I just sat there and cried.

I got out of the tub, wrapped in a towel, and sat on my bed holding a bottle of valium.

I didn't even know how many I'd have to take.

I just imagined myself drifting off into a blissful sleep.

I savored the calmness I imagined would be mine — the darkness finally gone.

These fantasies gave me brief moments of peace.

Instead, I took my prescribed medication.

I called my husband and let him know I was struggling again.
And I cried.

The guided meditations aren't helping this morning.
My heart is racing. I'm freezing and sweating at the same time.
My stomach is a mess.
I'm lying in bed as waves of terror and despair crash over me.

I hear my kids getting ready for school.
My door is locked— they can't see me like this.
I think of how much they need me and cry, because I wish they didn't.
It's a weight tying me to this world.
I can't escape.

My thoughts race. They're blurry and fast.
What kind of mom am I? Don't they deserve better?
My heart is pounding. I can't go to work like this.
I sit on the bed again and beg God to kill me.

I'm holding the pills again.
I'm sobbing.

Somehow, I manage to get the kids on the bus.
The thought crosses my mind that I may never see them again.

I go back inside.

I'll be late for work... again.

I put the bottle away.

I've taken my meds, knowing that one is addictive and the other may stop working over time.

I'm desperate.

Because medications work until they don't.

I feel better for a few weeks, and then I crash.

I've exercised. I've meditated. I've prayed.

I've challenged negative thoughts in therapy.

I've taken the pills — and not taken the pills.

I've talked to friends and family who offer well intentioned advice, but they don't really know.

I want to find joy in my life.

I love my family and friends.

I pray for strength.

And then I pray for death.

I am consumed by terror and despair.

My happy moments are stolen.

My future is filled with fear.

I continue to think about escape.

Somehow, I made it into the office that morning. But not long after that, I stopped going to work altogether.

Clearly, I was in a major depressive episode at the time, but I remember thinking these things. My mother-in-law started coming over in the mornings to take care of the kids while I lay in bed, under the covers, crying — desperately wanting a way out of the pain. Even just to sleep for a while. I would wallow in guilt and shame, hating myself for what I saw as weakness. Locked away in my room. And when I say hating myself, I mean HATE. I saw myself as useless and pathetic, honestly wondering how I could be so worthless. I was convinced that everyone else saw me that way, too. That kind of shame is unbearable. I remember the pain. Relentless. Suffocating. I write, but I can't find the words to really articulate what it felt like. It's one of those things you truly can't understand unless you've lived it. Looking back, I honestly believe I was under spiritual attack, and it almost killed me.

My moods were cyclical. Every morning, like clockwork, I would wake up in a full-blown panic, frozen with dread and self-loathing. I couldn't move; I'd just lie there, paralyzed. By early afternoon, my mood would stabilize enough that I could eat a piece of toast or something small. And by evening, I'd feel some hope, just a glimmer, that maybe things could change. It became so predictable that I started writing letters from my "night self" to my "morning self," to reassure her that she would be okay. But as time went on, the mornings stretched longer and longer, swallowing up more of the day.

When my kids were outside playing, I would watch them from my bedroom window: jumping on the trampoline, laughing, running around with the dogs in the backyard. Nothing was stopping me from going out there. Physically, I was fine. We were financially stable. I had a job I loved. There was no loss, no grief, no major crisis. Just me and my moods. Once again, facing a monster I couldn't see and didn't understand.

I started medication again alongside therapy, and for those of you who don't know what that process is like, imagine throwing a bunch of medicated darts at a target and praying one sticks without doing too much damage. That's basically it. There are meds for anxiety and depression, but they come with side effects and zero guarantees. The doctors come up with a "best guess" based on a few factors, but they'll straight up tell you they don't really *know*. My experience with medication was not a pleasant one. At first, I was prescribed an antidepressant that helped me sleep, which was a Godsend. For the first time in forever, I felt hope. I thought maybe this was all a chemical issue (just Clinical depression) and a pill could fix it. For about a week, I felt okay, maybe even good. But then — BAM — the morning panic returned. And this time, it felt even worse. I think mostly because I'd tasted hope again. Losing that was devastating.

We tried all sorts of medication cocktails. Some left me with horrible side effects. One caused insomnia, which created a bigger issue than what I started with. Another gave me facial tics. One even had the opposite effect, making my anxiety skyrocket. At one point, I was on five different medications — some just to counteract the side effects of the others. I was desperate. I stopped going to work and went on medical leave. My manager — God bless her — somehow made it so that I was paid in full for over a year while my disability retirement was being processed. That woman, Sara, was a blessing to me. I'll never forget her.

My first hospitalization happened in December of 2018. My husband's aunt called me and could hear the desperation in my voice. She came to the house and saw me in what she later described as an "awful state." I'd been laying in bed all day, crying. She worried I was on the edge of active suicidal ideation. I was already having passive thoughts — waiting to die. Not yet planning anything, but not caring if I woke up either. Overdose was my first thought. I envisioned the fear melting away as I drifted to sleep. I wrote in my journal about slicing my wrist, wondering if the pain and panic would seep out with the blood. I thought about walking to a bridge near my house and jumping. Or driving off the road. I never told her any of that, but she knew. She said she could hear it in my voice and see it in my face. I had given up.

She convinced my husband to take me to the hospital. I was admitted at Sibley Memorial soon after. The intake process at a psych hospital is the *least* trauma-informed thing I've ever experienced. You strip down so they can check for wounds, rashes, anything "wrong" with your body. I went through the motions, numb. It felt like just another intervention that would fail.

I met other people there — some depressed like me, others dealing with different illnesses like paranoia or schizophrenia. Everyone gets lumped together, but we formed our own little "illness cliques." Us depressed folks clung to the hope that something would show up in our blood work or scans to explain how we ended up like this. There was comfort in the shared experience, but hospitals don't really treat you. They start you on new meds, make sure you're not a danger to yourself or others, and then send you home. I cried the day I was discharged because I knew I was still very sick. My kids thought I was visiting my mother in West Virginia. When I came back, they were overjoyed to see me, but I felt nothing but sadness, knowing nothing had changed. I faked it as best as I could *for them*. I loved my children deeply; all I wanted was the best for them. As crazy as it seems, I believed that what was best for them was not me.

One day, it all became too much. I had on the sunglasses and took the kids to the bus stop. I watched them get on the bus and decided I couldn't take it anymore. I needed relief. I went inside and took a bunch of pills. I don't remember what or how many. I just wanted to sleep one way or another. By then, every time the bus pulled away, I'd already begun to think, *what if this is the last time I see them?* The rest of that day is a blur. I have brief memories of arguing with EMS in my bedroom. The next thing I remember is waking up the next morning, confused, with electrodes stuck to my chest. It was my daughter's fifth-grade graduation. I showered, peeled off the stickers without really thinking, and kept moving.

I later found out my mother-in-law had discovered me unresponsive and called 911. I'd taken a dangerous dose of benzodiazepines — the electrodes had been used to monitor my heart and vitals. Apparently, I spoke to a psychiatrist at the hospital who concluded it was an accidental overdose, so I was discharged. I had no memory of these events. Even the next day was hazy. I remember taking pictures at my daughter's graduation, but not being very present. I know I enjoyed the feeling of numbness. That's all.

My friend Debbie recently filled in more of the gaps for me. She said I had texted her a string of random letters and symbols. When she couldn't get hold of me, she called my mother-in-law — just as EMS arrived. I was being "uncooperative," and they told her if I didn't go willingly, the police would assist. That's what got me to go. That was enough to convince me to go. My sister visited me at the hospital and said I acted "drunk," showing off pictures of my children and laughing a lot. I'm glad I don't remember that.

My friends and family were there. I was surrounded by people who cared. But even with all the support, I could not get out of the depths of my despair. Debbie, my best friend to this day, was especially supportive. Somehow, she gets me and has always "gotten me." Even when I go silent for months, she gives me the space and grace to do so, knowing that I will come back when I am ready. And I always do.

After the overdose, the hospital recommended that someone stay with me, but shortly after, I was alone again. My husband took my daughter to softball and brought my son — probably afraid to leave him alone with me. He *tried*. He hid my meds, took my car keys, and only left for short periods. But he didn't know how sick I really was. As soon as they left, my altered brain took over. I found a hidden set of keys to our older car, drove to the store, and bought a bottle of Unisom. I went back home and took almost the entire thing. People ask if that was a suicide attempt, and my honest answer is that I don't really know. I didn't intentionally desire death; I desired relief. I wanted the pain to stop. But I had already convinced myself that if something *did* happen to me, maybe it was for the best.

People view suicide as selfish, and it is. The pain goes away for you (depending on your religious beliefs), but you pass it on to everyone who loves you. At the time, though, that is not what you think. I wasn't in a rational state of mind. In my mind, I would have been doing everyone a favor by releasing them from the burden of me. That's how depression lies to you. It tells you that you're worthless, that your absence would be a gift. I believed my kids deserved a better mom. I believed my husband would eventually remarry someone stronger, more capable. I believed God would understand — maybe this was what He had planned all along. I felt like God had gone silent as I suffered.

I woke up to my husband shaking me with the empty Unisom box in his hands. He was furious, asking me why I kept doing this when I had children and people who loved me. I had no answer. I hated myself more than ever. And to my surprise, the overdose didn't work as I'd expected. I didn't fall into a blissful dreamland of sleep. Instead, my legs turned to jelly, my hands shook uncontrollably, and my pupils were blown wide. I looked possessed. In that moment, I saw something in myself that terrified me. A demon. Sure, maybe I was hallucinating—that happens with an overdose — but it was enough to scare me. I was scared of death, of hell, everything.

A little later, I looked at pictures of my kids in the living room. I contemplated never seeing them again and realized I wanted to live, just not like *this*. By then, my husband had gone to bed. I tried to reach out for help, but when I looked at my phone, the numbers looked like random symbols I couldn't read. Unable to dial anyone, I sat there and waited, praying I wouldn't die.

The next thing I remember is Debbie showing up at my house. Apparently, I sent something that night. Nothing coherent, but when she read it the next morning, it was enough to make her come over to my house. She saw me. She saw the bottle. Saw everything, and took me back to the hospital. They called it a suicide attempt this time. That was probably the worst day of my life, the lowest point I had ever been. I didn't think it was possible, but I hated myself even more.

Debbie brought me a necklace of a butterfly made from a semicolon. The charm read: "fighter." I didn't wear it because I didn't feel like one. But I keep it in my charm bowl from Israel. One day, when I'm ready to tell this whole story out loud, I'll wear it. Maybe then I'll feel like I've earned it. But at that point, I didn't feel like I deserved it. My mental struggles consumed me, and I didn't yet see a hopeful way out.

Below is what my psychologist wrote in a progress note for my employer:

"Patient has made minimal improvements and continues to experience ongoing symptoms related to her diagnosis."

"Patients' symptoms interfere with her daily functioning and employment."

"Patient prognosis is guarded."

"Patient experiences panic, anxiety, and depression symptoms daily and has had minimal improvement".

"Patient is totally incapacitated from her mental health diagnosis, in excess of twelve months, due to debilitating symptoms of depression, anxiety, and post-traumatic stress disorder."

HISTORY:

Patient is a 41 year old female who has experienced recurrent symptoms of Major Depression, Panic Disorder and Post Traumatic Stress Disorder. Patient was hospitalized in December of 2017 at Sibley Memorial Hospital. Subsequently patient was referred to and participated in the Partial Hospitalization Program at St. Mary's Hospital. Ms. Cross attended the program from 12/28/2017 to 2/6/2018. She showed minimal improvement, however she continued to experience continued symptoms of Panic Disorder, Major Depression and Post Traumatic Stress Disorder. Patient returned to the partial program on 2/26/18 – 3/7/2018. Patient transitioned to outpatient services and began seeing a Psychiatrist, Dr. Harry Gill, on an outpatient basis on May 1, 2018. Patient was hospitalized at St. Mary's Hospital on two occasions for suicidal attempts. June 12 – 15, 2018 and June 15 – 19, 2018). Patient began seeing a psychologist, Dr. Raquel Gordon on June 27, 2017. Patient is currently being treated for intensive trauma based therapy. Patient has made minimal improvements and continues to experience ongoing symptoms related to her diagnoses. . Patients' symptoms interfere with her daily functioning and employment. Patient is not able to return to her current employment. Patient prognosis is guarded

DIAGNOSIS:
F41.01 Panic Disorder
F33.2 Major Depressive Disorder, recurrent, severe without psychotic features
F43.12 Post Traumatic Stress Disorder, Chronic

TREATMENT AND RESPONSE:

Patient experiences panic, anxiety and depression symptoms daily and has had minimally improvement.

PROGNOSIS:

Patient's prognosis is guarded.

Patient is totally incapacitated from her mental health diagnosis, in excess of 12 months due to debilitating symptoms of depression, panic and post traumatic stress disorder

I finally allowed my family to know what was going on. Suddenly, my siblings and my father were at the hospital. The fear of being found out began to fade in the warmth of their support. For the first time in a long while, I felt loved. I think that was the beginning of a turning point — a small spark of hope. I had always been terrified of becoming like my mother — unable to care for myself — and in that moment, I saw myself as exactly that. But I also saw something else: I wasn't alone. My family was still there, showing up for me. I had built a narrative in my head that my husband wouldn't — couldn't — take care of me. Why should he? Why should anyone? What I believed about myself — that I was a burden — I projected onto him. I told myself that he stayed only because it would look bad if he didn't. After all, who leaves their very sick wife? His indifference and, at times, coldness reinforced my beliefs. What I couldn't see then was that he was breaking under the weight of my instability. While I was unraveling, he was holding up everything else: our home, our children, our lives. He was silently preparing for a reality where I might never recover. He was scared and lost. And he didn't know what to do.

Today, he can admit that he made mistakes. He's told me he didn't know how to support me when I needed it most. We've since talked about how fear and sadness show up in him as anger — one of the few emotions he was ever allowed to express growing up. Back then, his reactions were limited: either he got angry or he withdrew, hoping things would somehow fix themselves. He still had to live life while I was in crisis. The kids had school and activities. Bills had to be paid. Life had to go on. Did he do everything right? No. He'd be the first to admit it. But he stayed and hoped things would get better.

During this time, he achieved one of his biggest successes in his professional career, but he never got to celebrate it. My crisis swallowed everything. He once told me that all he could think about was how to keep the family afloat while the rest of our world crumbled. To him, his success was just that, a way to keep us financially stable — rather than a personal celebration. Looking back, I'm sure he felt robbed of that moment, even though he's never said it aloud.

This time, I was hospitalized at St. Mary's. The director of the program happened to be a friend of my husband's — our daughters played softball together. I was mortified that my pain and shame were now visible to people in our everyday life. I'm sure my husband felt the same. One of the therapists was an intern I had once helped train. She kindly avoided interacting with me, which I appreciated. Professionally, she couldn't have engaged with me anyway, but the weight of how far I'd fallen hit hard in that moment. I stayed at St. Mary's for a week and left with a new diagnosis and new medication, but it was, once again, more about stabilization than true healing. They release you once you're no longer a danger to yourself or others. But something meaningful did come from that stay: I stopped hiding from my family.

My dad became one of my biggest supporters. He would come to my house and sit with me in silence, letting me know he didn't have the answers, but that he would love me while we figured it out. Sometimes I went to his house just to be near him. I don't think I had ever truly felt unconditionally loved by anyone in my life other than my mother and grandmother until then. By this time, my grandmother had passed, and my mother was too sick to be present. My dad filled that space in a way I didn't expect. He made me feel safe just by being there.

Two of my sisters, my friend Debbie, my sister-in-law, and both of my in-laws also offered support in their own ways. My stepfather, unexpectedly, became a kind and understanding outlet. As a combat veteran, he knew dark places. Our experiences were obviously different, but we shared some similar struggles. I also learned that my older brother had suffered with a panic disorder in his twenties and had struggled for years. It's amazing what you discover when you let people in. I realized that more people than I imagined could relate — even if only a little. And those who couldn't showed up anyway. No one judged or criticized me. Instead, some comforted me. Some helped with the day-to-day. And others pushed me forward when I wanted to give up.

I let It Grow

Chapter 6

The Separation

When I was hospitalized the first time, I would not allow my husband to tell anyone. But after the second hospitalization, he decided he could no longer keep this secret for me. I was so terrified of the potential rejection and humiliation that it didn't occur to me that by keeping this secret, I was also preventing him from receiving the support he needed. I don't know why I suffered in silence for so long. My fears weren't rooted in reality; they were projections of my own self-loathing onto the world around me. And even if those fears turned out to be true, reality would have been far kinder than the horror I created in my mind.

When I returned home, I was still very sick. But I decided I was going to fight and not give up. I would no longer entertain thoughts of escape through medication or self-harm — and since that day, I haven't. I moved into an empty bedroom upstairs — honestly, I had considered not returning home at all, but I couldn't bear the thought of leaving my children — and I completely shut myself off from my husband. I no longer trusted him. In my eyes, he had failed me. I never communicated any of this to him; I simply made the quiet decision to regain my independence and eventually leave. I was so angry at him for his inability to express love, compassion, concern, or empathy. Why did I have to seek emotional support from my dad, my siblings, and friends? Why couldn't my own husband be what I needed?

Even as I wrestled with anxiety and depression, new symptoms started to emerge. I couldn't escape my genetic wiring or childhood trauma. As I mentioned earlier, I had always lived with OCD symptoms: orderliness, list-making, checking, and ruminating. While it affected my quality of life, I had grown so used to it. It just felt like a part of who I was, rather than a disorder. And maybe it still is, even though the symptoms are much less severe today. Before this time, I had never researched OCD. I knew some people had it "bad" — like handwashing or checking things excessively — but I didn't see my habits as falling into that category. I was too focused on my "real" issues: anxiety and depression.

Around this time, I also suffered an ectopic pregnancy. I'd been experiencing a lot of pain and discomfort that I brushed off until it became severe enough that I fainted. My husband, thankfully home at the time, rushed me to the hospital. They discovered I was bleeding internally and performed emergency surgery. Physically, I recovered well, except for one thing: a persistent high-pitched ringing in my ears. Tinnitus. It was constant. During the day, background noise helped, but at night, it was unbearable. I tried everything, including pillows, fans, and white noise machines, but I struggled to sleep. I believe the combination of hormonal shifts and this ongoing physical distress contributed to what came next.

Seemingly out of the blue, I started having intrusive thoughts about contamination and infectious diseases. The first thought came to me while I was participating in a partial hospitalization program. Each day, I would pass by medical staff in scrubs, gowns, and masks. Suddenly, I felt exposed and vulnerable. Why was I walking around unprotected? Around the same time, my son contracted a pretty nasty case of pink eye, which I also caught. No matter how many medications we tried, it kept coming back. And what started out as a relatively minor illness became a full-blown obsession overnight. I began to worry about losing my eyesight or developing other illnesses. And I would search endlessly on Google for reassurance, just to fall deeper into panic as I fixated on rare worst-case outcomes, I was sure I had. I became paranoid. I feared contracting herpes in the eye from a kiss. I started using my shirt to open doors and wore gloves at the gas pump. I spiraled into all these compulsive behaviors to avoid contamination. My anxiety heightened, and although rationally I knew none of it made sense, I couldn't stop.

Then came the darkest thoughts that I told no one. They were terrifying and repulsive. One day, I was driving in a relatively decent mood when I saw a group of children waiting at a bus stop. A thought barged into my mind: *What if you just swerved into them and ran them all over?"* I was horrified. My heart raced. Where had that come from? What was wrong with me? Another thought soon followed: *"What if you're crazy, like Andrea Yates, and one day you kill your own children?"* I had never had any desire or intent to hurt anyone — especially not my children. That's what made the thoughts so unbearable. They didn't feel like mine. I felt possessed by a mind I no longer recognized.

Desperate to understand, I began researching women who killed their children to convince myself I wasn't like them. I became hypervigilant. I avoided knives and refused to be with my kids alone. I remember one morning my son slept in later than usual, and I panicked — *"Did I kill him and not remember?"* The fear was so visceral, I couldn't breathe. It started to feel like I was living in a nightmare. I couldn't eat or sleep. The thoughts wouldn't stop, and no amount of reassurance was enough. Because there's no way to prove with 100% accuracy that you won't go crazy and hurt someone. It's just something you know... until one day you don't. I couldn't bear the weight of that uncertainty.

I finally googled something helpful and found out that all of my recent thoughts about contamination, disease, and harm were different forms of OCD. What a relief it was to have a name for it. But learning it was "just OCD" didn't make it disappear. OCD thrives on doubt and demands certainty, and I couldn't be certain that it was *just* OCD. I knew I needed help. After researching, I found the OCD and Anxiety Center in Wisconsin, a residential program that specializes in OCD and co-occurring conditions like anxiety and depression. I knew I had to go. But leaving was incredibly hard.

This wasn't a short trip. I live in Maryland, and the program would keep me away for nearly two months. From the day after Halloween until just before Christmas, I wouldn't be able to see my kids. I worried about the little things I would miss, like who would decorate the house? Or set up the tree? And move our elf-on-the-shelf, Ginger Sparkle Toes? I know those things may seem trivial given everything, but they were real emotional barriers for me. I had tried so hard to be a good mom despite my struggles. One of my biggest regrets is how my mental health affected my ability to be present. But the elf? I nailed that. She didn't just move around; she caused mischief, left notes, brought gifts, and fixed toys. Once, for example, she crashed a Barbie car; another time she drank all of our syrup; and a different time she repaired my daughter's toy horse's broken leg. She meant a lot to the kids. In fact, I still have letters they wrote to her. I hold onto those memories when the guilt creeps in. Proof I got some things right.

I left for the OCD program on November 1st. The night before, my husband and I took the kids out trick-or-treating. They knew I was going somewhere to get better, so I wouldn't be sad all the time. That night, we met my sister at Panera.

I was staying with her, and she would take me to the airport the next morning. Saying goodbye to my kids was brutal. They cried. I cried. I hated myself. Why couldn't I just be normal? Why did I have to cause so much pain?

The first week at the center, I barely left my bed. I cried constantly. I couldn't eat or sleep. I missed my kids, and I was overwhelmed by intrusive thoughts that terrified me day in and day out. I believed I was going crazy, that maybe this wasn't OCD after all (a common OCD fear, ironically). And if it *was* OCD, I was sure I had the worst possible version. But I wasn't alone in that. If you can believe it, there were other people in the program who had more severe presentations than I did. There was a young woman who couldn't get to the bathroom and soiled herself because she had to walk "just right." Another man would take days to leave his room because he was "stuck." And others bathed or washed their hands for hours at a time. While my symptoms weren't as visible, they were just as consuming. I was once labeled "Pure O" — purely obsessional OCD — because I didn't have obvious compulsions. But I did have them: seeking reassurance, researching endlessly, avoiding triggers.

OCD is a cycle. You have some type of obsessive fear that causes anxiety, and a compulsion (even mental ones like researching or repeating thoughts) temporarily relieves it. One of my biggest obsessions was the fear that I would harm my children — what's known as "harm OCD." I couldn't stop thinking I was capable of it. My compulsions were to ask people if I was "crazy," research how people knew they wouldn't hurt their kids, and look up late-onset schizophrenia. But relief never lasted.

Another interesting thing about OCD is that it isn't limited to a single fear. When one obsession fades, another surfaces, like a game of whack-a-mole. This is why treatment has to be so targeted. The most effective form of treatment for OCD is Exposure and Response (or ritual) Prevention. It involves facing your fear head-on without engaging in the compulsion. My friends with contamination fears, for example would be exposed to things that would trigger their fears, like touching a door knob. They were then prevented from washing their hands and asked to sit and monitor their anxiety. We were all given stopwatches to see how long it took our anxiety to decrease from its peak to its eventual end, until we learned that the anxiety *would* pass without the ritual. And more importantly, the feared consequence never actually happened.

I had to do my own terrifying exposures. One assignment involved reading about mothers who killed their children — something I had avoided obsessively. I had to think about what I might have in common with them and write stories where my worst fears came true. No reassurance. No researching. No avoidance. The goal was to stare down the very thing I feared most.

The variety of the exposures in the program were often a source of laughter for us. One very specific form of OCD harm is the fear of yelling or saying something terribly offensive. The exposure, of course, was to yell things at staff, who would respond in ways designed to heighten discomfort. We shared our obsessions and compulsions openly and supported each other through the process. There was great comfort in talking with other people who shared this bizarre disorder. We laughed, we cried, and we rooted for one another. Some people couldn't finish treatment because it was too overwhelming. But for those who stayed, the work made a difference.

I also participated in a research study using an app for exposures. I submitted a list of trigger words — like "lunatic," "insane," and "murderer" — and neutral words like "table" or "lampshade." The words flashed randomly on the screen, and I tapped a button when I saw them. It seemed simple, but over time, I reacted less intensely to the trigger words. I think it helped. And yes, I appreciated the gift cards for participating. One of the most powerful exposures was inducing a panic attack on purpose. Panic attacks used to terrify me. I'd worry about having one. I'd worry about dying. I'd even been to the ER more than once, convinced I was having a full-blown heart attack due to the intense feeling they produce. These were the symptoms:

- Rapid heart rate
- Hyperventilating - feeling unable to catch my breath
- Dizziness
- Legs felt like jelly
- Light-headed
- Fears that I was going to die
- Cold flashes
- Numbness

To confront this, I had to recreate the symptoms. I ran stairs, breathed through a straw, spun in a chair — anything to trigger the panic. At first, it was awful. But with repetition, my body stopped reacting so intensely. Eventually, the panic attacks stopped altogether. At any time in the OCD center, you could walk in and see us spinning in chairs, yelling obscenities, researching horrific crimes, sitting in a dark room, or touching doorknobs. To an outsider, it would look bizarre. But to us, it was healing. The biggest lesson I learned was the absolute need to face discomfort. Avoidance only feeds fear. I learned that lesson, and am still practicing it every day.

Medication was also part of my recovery. I don't know how it works, and honestly, most psychiatrists can't fully explain it either. But at that time, it was essential. It seemed to slow my thoughts enough that therapy could actually work. The combination of therapy and medication has now helped me move in the right direction. I stayed on medication for about two years after the program.

While I was in treatment, my husband visited me. He sent flowers on our anniversary. He took care of the kids and made sure I spoke to them every night. We texted daily. But despite everything I was learning about confronting fear and avoiding avoidance, I still couldn't open up to him. I went through the motions, but I couldn't have the conversations I really needed to have. Too much was left unsaid.

When I returned home after treatment, my thoughts and feelings towards my husband hadn't changed. I still felt emotionally disconnected and unable to trust him. I carried what I call "righteous anger." Every therapist I shared my story with affirmed that my husband was not only avoidant, but also emotionally abusive and neglectful. Of course, what I shared was the worst of his behavior. I researched online, and the internet offered no shortage of validation. I read article after article that supported what I wanted to believe: that he was emotionally incapable, perhaps a narcissist, maybe even a psychopath. The symptoms matched just enough to feel convincing. And when the consensus in those spaces was, "Leave — these people don't change," I clung to that advice. I didn't leave room for growth or healing. I didn't focus on repairing the relationship. I focused on starting over without him.

The emotional divide between us only deepened. I continued to position myself and the kids against him, often unconsciously. And in response, he remained angry and defensive — his default reaction — which only confirmed the narrative I had built: that he was incapable of change, empathy, or connection.

In February 2023, I made my move.

Chapter 7

Reflections

It's telling what you choose to take with you and what you leave behind when you're starting over. For me, it was the over 30 photo albums, carefully arranged in chronological order, documenting a lifetime with my kids. I've always been intentional about capturing memories. Each of my children has a fully detailed baby book — pages of journals and letters I wrote in an effort to hold onto the fleeting moments of their childhood. I took every one of those books with me. They were proof. Proof that I showed up, that I tried, that I was there. As I've said before, my greatest regret is all the time I lost being sick and afraid. I was determined not to lose any more. But my kids weren't little anymore. The window to recreate the childhood I'd always imagined for them had closed. Some things can't be redone. You don't get do-overs with people.

My daughter, sixteen at the time, was struggling with her own anxiety, panic, and school avoidance. I supported her as best I could, though she naturally preferred spending most of her time with friends. My son had just started high school and was more interested in video games than anything else. They had their own lives, and I had mine. I threw myself into work, taking on new leadership roles and responsibilities that consumed most of my energy. It kept me from dwelling on the past or worrying too much about the future. Work was the perfect distraction. Whenever loneliness crept in, I stayed too busy to let it take root. Without even realizing it, I was building a life centered on avoidance. And the problem with avoidance is — it doesn't last. You can't always be busy. Inevitably, still moments come. And when they did, the emotions hit like a flood. Raw. Fresh. Unrelenting. I didn't want to feel them. I had made my decision. I was moving on. Life was supposed to be better now. But the truth was, I hadn't done the work. I hadn't really looked at myself or my patterns. I believed that once I got out of that house — out of that marriage — everything would just fall into place. I had convinced myself that everything in that life was toxic. And yes, there were bad times, painful times. But I hadn't prepared for how much I'd miss the good ones. The first major holiday I spent alone forced a realization I wasn't ready for: maybe, just maybe, part of all this was me.

One thing that my dedication to work brought me was financial stability. In time, I felt ready to put down roots. I thought maybe that was what I needed to feel settled, safe, and secure. In March, I bought a house. There was a white squirrel living in the woods near the property. White squirrels are rare in the area where I live in Southern Maryland. They're said to bring good luck or to signal change, and the need to prepare for it. They survive despite standing out — bold and vulnerable without the camouflage of their brown counterparts. All signs pointed to my growth and the house being the new direction I needed. Six months later, the squirrel was gone... I never really believed in signs anyway.

Around that time, I listened to a podcast by Jordan Peterson, where he offered strategies for managing depression and anxiety. One idea in particular stuck with me: the need to start with the simple acknowledgment — "I am miserable"— and to examine what that truly means in the context of your life. He posed a question that struck me hard: *Am I depressed, or is my life just awful?* I sat with that and began to assess specific areas of my life:

- Intimate relationships
- Friendships
- Career
- Education and lifelong learning
- Resistance to temptation
- Self-care
- Community

I began to think seriously about what needed to change, because the honest answer was: *my life is just awful*. And the reality of that was that it was, at least in part, my fault.

I started therapy again with a new therapist who introduced me to a different approach to healing and recovery. She challenged me to look inward and take accountability for the role I played in my own suffering. After all, the only person I could truly change was myself. She didn't see me as a victim, and because of that, I began to see myself as the capable grown woman I was. I started to believe I could choose happiness over sadness. Forgiveness over bitterness and resentment. I could choose *my* story, rather than letting others tell me how I should think, feel, or act.

It was alarming to realize that I didn't even know what I wanted in so many areas of my life: in friendships, in family relationships, in my marriage. If I didn't know what I wanted, how could I communicate it to anyone else? How could I work toward goals or dreams that weren't even clear to me? Yes, I wanted safety, but I wanted more than that. Safety can get in the way of *living*. Living requires risk, and the two greatest risks I avoided were abandonment and rejection. But if you avoid those, you also miss out on a true connection. Anything of value requires effort and the risk of loss. My whole life, I had hidden from people truly knowing or caring about me because I was terrified of rejection. I also refused to depend on others—fiercely clinging to my independence and autonomy — because I was equally terrified of abandonment. Keeping people at arm's length felt "safe," but it also kept me very, very lonely. Comfort can be deceptive; sometimes it's a trick that prevents you from feeling the discomfort necessary for growth.

So, what do I want? I am still working on that part. But I *do* know what I no longer want: to be limited by my fears. I'm exhausted from running. I had to look at myself honestly and begin trusting my thoughts and feelings. I needed to figure out how to end my own suffering. On the outside, once again, I looked successful. I had left a destructive marriage. I had a great career and even bought my own home. But nobody really *knew* me. I was lonely, even though people told me I was strong. I was sad while people said I was successful. It was a contradiction that I lived with every day. I was doing what I was supposed to do — what people expected me to do — but none of it felt right. It's easy for others to steer your life when they don't have to live with the consequences. And I let them. But if I wanted things to change, I had to take the reins. I had to figure out what *I* needed and wanted—and that was something I had never really done before.

One of the first decisions I made was to prioritize my physical well-being. I changed my diet to nurture my body and started exercising regularly. I made a point to show up for myself every day. Six months later, I was down twenty pounds, and my mood and outlook had significantly improved. During this time, I stayed in therapy and journaled, doing the hard internal work of figuring myself out. I also began to search for purpose. I wanted to do something meaningful. So, I began fostering elderly dogs — and somehow, I ended up adopting two: Buttercup, a 13-year-old Shih Tzu, and Dolly, a 9-year-old Lab. I also took in a 1-year-old cat named Jack. My animals brought me comfort and companionship.

This time, I wasn't avoiding my feelings. And when I started to fall back into old patterns, my therapist called me out. It was hard to sit with the truth of where I was. I was forty-seven, on the brink of divorce, anxious, and lonely. But I was facing it — really facing it — for the first time. And let me tell you: facing your emotions is *hard*. Especially when they feel like a tsunami. I don't know if it's genetic, learned, or rooted in trauma, but anxiety — and to a lesser extent, depression — has always been part of my life. Even when things seem stable, there's an undercurrent of dread, a fear that something bad is coming. This is especially true when something throws a wrench in my day-to-day life. If I get sick or a financial issue pops up, I struggle to cope. I'm afraid the big problems will come back — and when they do, I'll be alone and unable to manage them. There's still a little girl inside me who's terrified of being abandoned. The crazy thing is, people *do* reach out to me — friends, family — but I routinely ignore them. It's the classic push-pull of avoidant attachment. What I want, I'm afraid to have.

During our separation, my husband made attempts to reconcile. We went on dates, but they felt forced. During our separation, my husband made efforts to reconcile. We went on dates, but they felt forced. We weren't having real conversations. By unspoken agreement and years of dysfunction, we slid right back into our old roles, pretending everything was fine. He thought the dates meant we were moving toward reconciliation. I felt they confirmed we had no future together. We were living in two different realities.

When I bought my house in March, that was the wake-up call he needed. I texted him to say I had filed for divorce and retained a lawyer. I believed it was the best decision for all of us. I surrounded myself with people who agreed. But here's the part I don't talk about as clearly, at least not yet:

my own destructive patterns. It's easy to see myself as a kind person. And in many ways, I *am.* But under certain conditions, I can be pretty darn evil, too. I judge myself by my *intentions*, while judging others by their *actions.* It's a convenient way to dodge accountability.

I described how I created a triangulation in the family — myself and the kids, versus him. We disagreed on some fundamental parenting issues that felt threatening to me. I pretended to be passive, but I wasn't. I had no real boundaries with our children, especially the two oldest. Like my mother, I tried to protect them from everything. My intentions were good, but in the long run, that kind of parenting is not effective. You can't just love your kids; you have to guide them, too. My husband went the other route. He was a stern and strict disciplinarian. With his harsh parenting, he contributed to the triangulation just as much as I did. Naturally, the kids gravitated toward my warmth. I'll never forget a scholarship essay my son wrote. The prompt asked which historical figure he'd like to spend a day with. Most kids probably chose Jesus or a famous leader. My son wrote about wanting to meet his father *as a child*, to see who he was before he became so angry. He won that scholarship. If both of us had moved a little more to the center and agreed on how to raise our kids, I think many of the challenges we all face today could have been avoided.

I was also intentionally cold and cruel to him at times. used the silent treatment to punish him. I refused to acknowledge his accomplishments or interests. He'd ask me to join him for outings, errands, or events — and I'd say no, over and over again, just to hurt him. I couldn't directly address the conflict, so I fought with emotional withdrawal and passive aggression. People have told me, "That was just your trauma response." And maybe that's true — but does that make it right? I still made choices. I could have chosen differently. It wasn't just the reaction of a wounded victim. I know this because I've repeated this behavior in every relationship I've ever had.

Lately, I've been listening to Jordan Peterson. In one of his talks on marriage, he says something like: *Your partner might be a snake — but you're no saint either.*

That line hit me. Hard.

In April, I received a message from my husband. It was heartfelt and apologetic, an honest attempt to take responsibility. In a last-ditch effort to save our marriage, he was vulnerable, expressing a willingness to go to counseling, to do *anything* that might give us one last chance. From his perspective, our recent dates had been going well. He believed he was giving me space to heal, that he wasn't rushing anything. He thought we still had time. I thought we were only delaying the inevitable. After nearly 50 years of thinking, feeling, and behaving a certain way, change felt impossible. I didn't believe he was even open to trying. Reading his message was difficult — it didn't align with the narrative I'd created about him. From the beginning of our separation, I prayed for a miracle, for reconciliation. But if I'm honest, I didn't truly believe he could change. And yet… he didn't "move on" as I'd expected. He mourned our absence. He agreed to therapy. He wanted to talk. I wasn't prepared for that. It had been easier to hold on to his worst moments and let them define him. Easier to keep him boxed in under the label of "narcissist," a label I had clung to far too tightly. So, I ignored his words. And I moved forward with the divorce.

At the same time, I was beginning, for the first time, to ask myself what *I* wanted and needed. That process was painful. It required honesty about where my choices had led me at 47, and what I needed to take responsibility for to create the life I wanted. I resigned from my role directing the clinical program and took a position providing direct care again. And when I sat with myself, I realized I was lonely. I began to see how my patterns had developed over time, how they affected me and my relationships, and, more importantly, what I wanted to do about it. It was freeing to realize that I had the power to make those changes. I reread his email over and over again. Was he truly willing and able to change? Or was I just lonely and vulnerable? I didn't respond. I kept my distance.

Then came the day we met on Zoom with our lawyers to discuss how to appraise the house and divide assets. It was the first time I had seen him in months. He looked different. He said he didn't want the divorce, but he knew I did — and he was willing to cooperate. He looked defeated. And my heart stirred. The only way I can describe it is that God moved me. We agreed to meet later that week at our favorite restaurant to talk — just the two of us, no lawyers. When we met, I saw a man I almost didn't recognize. He was in tears and spoke about what he wished he had done differently. He shared his remorse and a commitment to change, which was evident in the raw emotional vulnerability I had never seen from him before. We talked for three hours that night, finally saying the things we had left unsaid for years. Nearly two decades of marriage spilled out in one evening.

I left that night unsure of how to move forward. For the past year and a half, I had been moving down the path of divorce, adjusting to single motherhood. It felt like I was on a train I couldn't stop. I had plans for the divorce settlement — to pay off the home I had just bought. My friends had celebrated my "single womanhood." My family had come to terms with my new identity as a divorcée. My kids had adjusted. How do you just change your mind?

Well... maybe you don't have to. Perhaps not everything has to be decided right now. A few weeks ago, we started marriage therapy. We're both working on our own individual growth. We also started going to church together again. Who knows what will happen next?

Some of you reading this might feel sorry for me. When I read back what I've written, I see plenty of painful, messy moments. But that's because I've chosen to focus on the hard parts — the experiences that shaped my beliefs — so I can better understand why I am the way I am. And build empathy, not just for myself, but for others as well. I believe we all hold the capacity for both good and bad. But whatever we nurture... that's what we become. And the beautiful thing? We can change our story at any time. We're not prisoners of our past or our pain. We can look in the mirror and say: "This isn't working for me."

It wasn't all bad — it never is, for any of us. I've had incredibly beautiful moments in my life, and I have qualities I'm deeply proud of. I don't buy into the idea that suffering makes us strong. What made me strong was the love I received from people who supported me in the midst of it. Part of my healing now is intentionally noticing the good. Recalling positive memories. Creating more of them.

These days, I spend time every morning meditating on gratitude and joy. Even on my hardest days, I find small moments that fill me with light. I feel genuine happiness and excitement over the little things. I marvel at the weather. I welcome the change of seasons. I plan cozy meals and scary movie nights. I enjoy soft, warm blankets. I don't envy or covet. I feel content with the life I've built in my little home. I was never drawn to consumerism or the "next shiny thing" anyway.

Now, for the first time, I'm learning how to build deep, emotional connections with others. I don't carry resentment — not for anyone in my past, and not for the people in my life today. I have three children who share my weird sense of humor. They are wonderful, kind humans. I have an old dog who hates everyone but me, and a younger one who loves everyone. Every morning, they greet me like it's the best day of their lives — and in some ways, it is. I'm grateful to be alive, to have something to look forward to each day. I'm excited for the future I'm building — most of the time. And I can acknowledge that I'm still a work in progress.

I believe those who have suffered deeply often have the deepest capacity for gratitude. I believe some of us are wired, by biology or environment, to feel more intensely. We hurt more, yes. But we also experience joy more vividly. When I laugh, I laugh loudly. I *feel* joy in my bones. There were moments when I wanted to die.

Today, I choose to really live.

Selected writings:

The difference between then and now,
is being scared — and doing it anyway.
Today, my behavior dictates my feelings.
My feelings do not dictate my behavior.

I think I may always find my happiness
In the happiness of others.
I just have to learn
to see
when their happiness
destroys me.

When did I learn to silence the voice in my head that screamed THIS IS NOT OK?

Keeping the peace
was always the way
I made the unacceptable
acceptable.

I am going to keep to myself for a while —
to protect my dreams.
Because I can't tell the difference
between good and evil
sometimes.

The thousand different ways I wish I had been...
stronger, wiser, better —
I guess I did the best I could
with what I had.
But I know that's still not enough.

Why is it that I still think
maybe
it was my fault?

I am afraid that if I share this
growing joy,
you'll find a way
to steal it

I try to fix people
who don't believe they are broken —
and let them convince me
that I'm the broken one
while they are breaking me.

What is it called when I cry
and you pretend not to hear me?

I have always tried to find safety
With unsafe people
You would think that,
by now,
it wouldn't scare me.

But when I wake up to the familiar feeling —
46 years of fear,
Memories —
I cannot move.

Sometimes,

I don't miss you.
I could erase it all
except
The parts I made
with the possibility of who
I thought you could be.

Why is it that I am
afraid,
alone,
ashamed —
when I look at the phone
and it's you calling?

I am still waiting for this (joy)
not to happen.
But
I am brave enough
today
to plan for it anyway.

REMINDER
The illusion of safety and love (lies)

Was more frightening
than the reality
of being alone

I want to sit on my grandmother's porch again,
Look at the stars with her,
and catch lightning bugs with my brother —
and let them go.
I want to listen to my mother read me books about mouse
families,
collect leaves,
drink Hush Puppies,
watch ice skating and Nature,
and eat my grandmother's roast and potatoes.

I want to return to *simple*.
I want to feel safe again.

I used to be ashamed of my wild, uncombed hair.
and dirty clothes.
But I am proud of that little girl now.
I wish she knew that.

At that time, I couldn't —
for a thousand reasons.
But now,
I can.

I may get up scared,
But I can still get up.
I may not be certain,
But I can still make a decision.
It may be hard,
But it's not impossible.
I have the resources (they didn't have)
to create my dreams.

I feel my mother and grandmother
Living in me —
rooting for me.

I cannot fail.
I will not quit.

About the Author

This is my first book, and I am excited to share it with all of you! This book is based on true events in my life, family history, my own therapy journey, and my knowledge as a licensed therapist. I plan to continue writing as I have found it to be a helpful outlet for not only my feelings but also the creativity I have buried for so long. My passions in life, outside of work and family, include volunteering at my local animal shelter, especially with the senior dogs, playing card games, gardening, going to the movies, and true crime TV.

www.ingramcontent.com/pod-product-compliance
Lightning Source LLC
Chambersburg PA
CBHW052119030426
42335CB00025B/3052